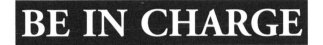

BE IN CHARGE

A LEADERSHIP MANUAL

How to Stay on Top

BE IN CHARGE

A LEADERSHIP MANUAL

How to Stay on Top

Alexander R. Margulis

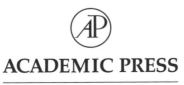

ACADEMIC PRESS

An imprint of Elsevier Science

Amsterdam   Boston   London   New York   Oxford   Paris
San Diego   San Francisco   Singapore   Sydney   Tokyo

Images copyright © Getty Images 2002.

This book is printed on acid-free paper.

Copyright © 2002, Elsevier Science (USA).

All Rights Reserved.
No part of this publication may be reproduced or transmitted in any form or by any means, electronic or mechanical, including photocopy, recording, or any information storage and retrieval system, without permission in writing from the publisher. Requests for permission to make copies of any part of the work should be mailed to: Permissions Department, Academic Press, 6277 Sea Harbor Drive, Orlando, Florida 32887–6777

Academic Press
An Elsevier Science Imprint
525 B Street, Suite 1900, San Diego, California 92101-4495, USA
http://www.academicpress.com

Academic Press
84 Theobolds Road, London WC1X 8RR, UK
http://www.academicpress.com

Library of Congress Catalog Card Number: 2002102528

International Standard Book Number: 0–12–471351–3

PRINTED IN THE UNITED STATES OF AMERICA
02 03 04 05 06 07 MM 9 8 7 6 5 4 3 2 1

Contents

To Hedi

Foreword

A lex Margulis is one of the great leaders in academic medicine. Evaluating his clinical expertise, I will leave to others. I would like to comment on the man and the leader.

Alex was the first in his field to reach out for new ideas. He embraced industry for technical collaboration. More importantly, he was open to any process idea that would make his department more competitive.

In addition, Alex was a great developer of people. He recognized the importance of leadership, something rare in healthcare. He gave his team time... cared about their development... and, ultimately, he created hundreds of disciplines.

I have had the opportunity to meet many great leaders. Alex is unique for his longevity, freshness of thought, and spirit. In his book, *Be in Charge: A Leadership Manual*, Alex shares these common sense views that can help us all.

Jeffrey R. Immelt

Preface

Speaking with colleagues in universities, mingling and observing the difficulties of heading business units, and recollecting my own difficulties, I became convinced that life could be made easier with a manual on how to cope.

This book is designed to provide some guidance through the thicket of problems encountered in handling people. While ways to successfully deal with situations in business and academia are often similar, the differences are most important, and with help I have tried to address them. There are many styles of leadership, but the truly successful chiefs work to gain respect, loyalty, and unstinted support from their associates and subordinates.

The manual also attempts to help women who have broken through the "glass ceiling" and become executives. There are not many of them, and while their number is increasing in the United States, they are still operating in a man's world.

My own experiences have been expanded through reading and particularly through interviews with many successful leaders. Although I am not quoting them directly, many of them will recognize their ideas.

I hope this manual will be helpful in managing the big and small problems that chiefs are encountering daily and are expected to solve. May their lives be easier after reading this manual.

Alexander R. Margulis

Acknowledgments

I am deeply grateful to all the authors of the books I have read and referenced. They contributed knowledge to what I have learned during my career. I have profited also from observing how leaders in business and academia operate. The individuals who consented to be interviewed and are listed at the end of this book have been invaluable. Without them, this opus would have been worthless. I am very much in debt to them for their time and help. I thank Dr. Susan Wall for reading the manuscript and giving me a sage critique. I have also had wise guidance, suggestions, and constructive criticism from my spouse, Dr. Hedvig Hricak. In short, I needed a lot of help.

WHAT IS LEADERSHIP?

A few basic rules can lead to success.

Leadership is the ability to inspire others to follow and change the future. Its basic ingredients are integrity, vision, courage, and loyalty to one's principles. The ability to lead is an innate quality that few people possess; those who wish to work for good causes hopefully will use this book. In general, leaders who leave the most memorable record are those who are highly ethical and do not practice in the mode that lofty ends justify all means. While some men and women are born with the ability to lead and inspire, these people are rare. However, most people can *learn* how to lead. The book is designed to provide the basic rules of how to be a successful leader.

As an introduction, here are a few of the basic rules. Do not strive to be loved. Go for respect and loyalty. Do not show your feelings in public except to inspire, and above all do not shout or, even worse, cry unless you have planned it in cold blood. Have genuine affection for your associates, feel profound loyalty for them. Pretending shows. Be a role model of hard work and modesty. Do not ask associates to work harder or longer than you do. Promise less than you deliver. Be approachable. Be generous with distributing titles, but make them meaningful. Delegate, but supervise. The leader is responsible for failures but should always share credit for successes. Your time is the most precious resource that you have. Budget it carefully and always prioritize. Women executives need to follow a few additional rules, some of which, regrettably, reflect our society's prejudices, and some result from physiologic gender differences. These will be dealt with in other chapters.

THE VARIOUS TYPES
OF CHIEFS

To succeed and advance, learn about the terrain and the people, have a consistent demeanor, and be aware that blood in the water attracts sharks. Remember that there is no job too big, there are only people lesser than the job.

Whether in business, government or academia, there are multiple levels of hierarchy, and each level has its own chief. As one ascends the staircase of the establishment's governance, each level is noted to have similar rules for success. As responsibilities increase, so do the number of associates and subordinates. The number of equals and superiors, however, decreases. Just as large amounts of money do not bring happiness but only more options, ascending the scale of hierarchy does not bring happiness, only a reduced number of people giving you orders. To be successful in the hierarchy and continue ascending the scales, one must realize that each governmental agency, company, or university, while generically similar to other such entities, has its own idiosyncratic identity. It is important to be familiar with that identity, as one's own behavior toward superiors, equals, or subordinates must be gauged accordingly.

Then there are regional peculiarities to consider. For instance for an executive in a company in New York to dress in a T-shirt and blue jeans would be considered very odd (except perhaps on an occasional Friday in certain companies that wish to emphasize togetherness and friendliness toward employees). This could be sufficiently eccentric for the region as to be considered unacceptable; conversely, it would be embraced as "in" among executives in Silicon Valley. In academia, however, dress depends on whether the executive is a laboratory scientist or one who deals with potential financial donors.

Dress and behavior are particularly important for women executives. While there may be regional differences, there, too, the rule should be as follows: Do not stick out. One should be conservative in a conservative environment. Do not be too avant-garde, ever, anywhere.

It is essential for a chief who is a candidate for promotion to higher levels to be proper, not to lead or participate in any revolutions, and not to bad-mouth his or her equals or superiors. Remember, as you ascend, you become highly quotable. A careless remark becomes interesting news and a source for gossip, and you can be quoted with malice (generally with distortion and out of context). Close friendships are a handicap except with clearly noncompeting equals. Otherwise they can lead to terrible disappointments and even generate enmities. Do not share your problems, and do not complain. Above all, do not show that you are hurt. Blood in the water attracts and excites sharks.

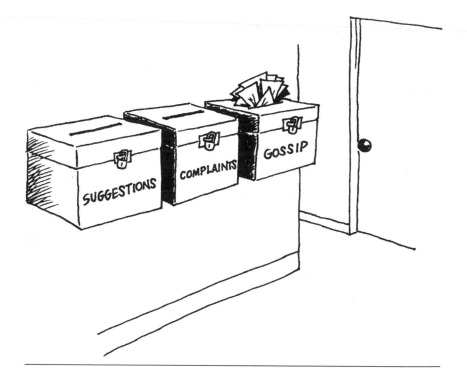

There are three styles of behavior for chiefs:

1. *The tyrant-dictator.* This leader creates many enemies who will be silent, wait for a slip, then attack. These enemies can be kept silent only by the continuous success of the leader. As success depends on

many factors, some of which the leader may have no ability to control, the tyrant-dictator leader must be both ruthless and lucky with enemies.

2. *The benevolent dictator.* This leader is friendly, considerate, courteous, and pleasant, but generally is liked and praised only as long as he or she is successful. In defeat, the benevolent chief will get no help and scant sympathy. Remember, the person on top has a lonely job. The benevolent dictator chief must be as ruthless with enemies as is the tyrant-dictator, but this leader must be less overt. For instance, the benevolent dictator would transfer an incompetent or undesirable employee with a good recommendation rather than fire.

3. *The chairman of the board.* Such a chief appoints committees but does not function as a true leader. Other people make the decisions, and he or she postures. Such chiefs often are humiliated in public by their very deputies. They may last a long time if the junta that backs him or her is able to share power among its members and uses the chief as a ceremonial figurehead.

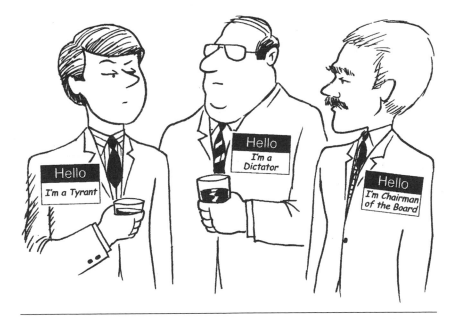

The secret for a successful chief is to delegate, supervise, never give up authority, and be consistent in order for the subordinates to know what to expect in a given situation. This creates respect and order. It is said that in armed forces units, chiefs with consistent behavior, whether tyrannical or considerate, are respected. Even the tyrant, if predictable, is accepted as "*our* son of a bitch."

In times of crisis, a successful chief is expected to act as a dictator (the title was given to a consul in times of danger by the senate of the Roman Republic), and his or her decisions (which in quiet periods would be challenged) are accepted without questions.

Generally, chiefs are not permanent fixtures. Some stay in the same position for the length of their career. Some move upward, often to their level of incompetence (Peter's principle). Others move laterally to the same level in another organization, out of desire for change. If such a move is suggested as a "lateral arabesque" (for instance, to an empty but impressive title as described in Peter's principle), this is the time to choose alternate employment or retire with dignity. For some, a move leads to a brilliant career. Although most executives, if the move is successful, credit this success to their perspicacity or unfailing instinct, the truth is that many factors are involved. The most important are timing, the general economic climate, and the state of well-being of the new organization. If it has been prosperous and well run by a former chief who was a business genius, one can predict lack of success for a protracted period unless the new chief is totally different, is his own man or woman, and never looks back. A less challenging opportunity arises when the new leader follows a miserable chief in an otherwise healthy environment that is waiting to reach its proper state of radiant health. The appointment to head a poor department in an otherwise successful company is most likely going to lead to success. Heading a great enterprise within a poor environment requires great skill to avoid being drawn down to the surrounding level. If everything is low in quality, including the branch, department, and the mother company or university, there must be compelling reasons for such a state of affairs. It is advisable for the new chief to study and attempt to find out why this situation exists. If there is a chance for overall improvement, this situation may lead to unimaginable success and upward mobility that will be combined with national and international recognition and visibility.

In the academic arena, an excellent example for the latter is what happened at the University of California, San Francisco (UCSF). Up to the mid-1960s, its medical school was an unexciting, private-practitioner-dominated, average-quality school. However, with the advent of jet planes making transcontinental flights, nonstop, affordable, and timely, recruitment to the West Coast was no longer akin to exile. With the key appointments of a few young, ambitious leaders from famous East

Coast universities and an emphasis on collegiality and team play, the quality of the University of California, Berkeley, was introduced to San Francisco. For a span of 10 years, every department recruited brilliantly from outside UCSF, creating an atmosphere of friendship and mutual loyalty like that of Camelot and the Knights of the Round Table. This Collegiality transformed the school into one of the national leaders of academic medical institutions.

To be a successful leader, whether in academia or in business, it is important to allow yourself free time to think. A successful leader should be involved with other activities unrelated to the job. It is important not to neglect one's own family, which should be a strong base of support, and also devote time to the betterment of the community in which one is living. Some executives complain that their jobs are so important that they do not have time for anything else. This restricts their outlook. Remember that there are truly no jobs so big as to fully absorb an individual. You must leave time for relaxation, reflection, and social obligations. Remember, there are no big jobs, there are only people who are less than the job they try to fill.

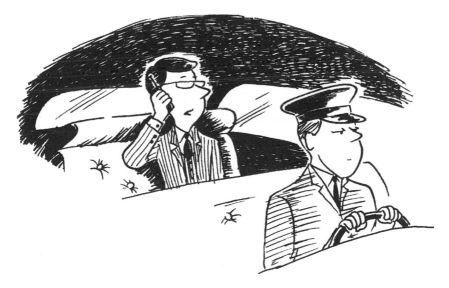

"... and they lived happily ever after. The end.
Now goodnight Billy. Daddy loves you very much."

GENDER DIFFERENCES:
Equal, but . . .

In a man's world, women should play by men's rules. Refuse to be intimated, but remember that chiefs don't cry.

There are laws against discrimination by gender, age, religion, sexual preference and so on regarding employment, treatment at work, promotion, and other factors. Many firms and universities have come to regret their indifference to obvious cases of sexual harassment, as well as discrimination in promotion and pay. It has cost them dearly, both financially and in adverse publicity. On the surface it would appear to the unsophisticated and personally uninvolved that gender discrimination is a matter of the, by now, long-gone insensitive and prejudiced past. The present, however, is much more complicated than the past, and it remains in a state of flux. To be fair, sexes are not equal. *Vive la différence!* First of all, career women (particularly in the United States) often must choose between total immersion in their career or having children, with the latter group devoting their time to the family. Even when a young woman has reached the top (which is uncommon for the young) and wishes to have or has children, it may be difficult for her to lead both a fully consuming career and a traditional family life. This is because emergencies will predictably happen in both areas of her life. Sometimes perimenopausal women must deal with the vicissitudes of hormonal fluctuations. This may, at times, temporarily or periodically affect a woman's outlook on life, as well as her interactions with colleagues and associates. Fits of anger or episodes of crying in meetings may confuse or blur her image as a strong leader. In this period of life, some women even struggle with depression. These symptoms generally are time limited and disappear once the physiology of menopause passes or is tempered with hormone replacement therapy. Some men at this age also go through an unsettling phase of life style change, defined by many as "male menopause." This is the stage when divorces, job changes, or even alcohol or drug addiction is frequent. However, many women as well as men sail through this time of life completely unbothered and find the experience liberating and energizing.

How does a woman reach the top and how does she stay there? It is a given that her intellectual and character qualities make her, at the very least, slightly better than her male competitors. What makes her reach the top are the following factors:

1. Consistent leadership behavior (vision, courage, integrity).
2. Absence of unfavorable publicity.
3. Good grooming and an inborn elegance. Most successful professional women (like men) understand that attention to appearance is important.
4. Powerful friends in influential positions
5. Perhaps most important, devoted and skillful mentoring. A mentor is a parent figure, someone who can criticize, suggest, analyze, advise, and be there to encourage or lend a shoulder to cry on. Good mentors are rare because they must be generous with time, forgiving, patient, wise and always available. If you have one, cherish him or her.

In our society, a woman executive cannot afford the same intimacies with associates that her male counterparts are allowed. She must be friendly, reserved, and somewhat distant, lest her behavior be misinterpreted. Men generally cannot forget that their colleague is a woman, and thus they behave differently with her than they do with a man.

While overt sexual harassment in the workplace has decreased, when it does exist, women often are reluctant to complain. They often try to ignore it, because of fear that a complaint or accusation may ruin their career. Even more often, they may not immediately recognize that sexual harassment is happening.

A much more subtle form of harassment is the flirtatious, joking, or suggestive approach that is full of compliments and can be interpreted in several ways. The best response is for the woman executive to ignore the flirtation, pretend not to grasp the implications, and just proceed normally as if no advances have been made. If that does not help, a short, but a definitive "Cut it out" almost always serves as a successful retort. The woman executive can pretend (overtly) to make notation of the date and time with "there you go again." Many men are still uncomfortable reporting to a female chief. When a woman reaches the top, expectations are different, and many of the subordinates feel the need to test her mettle. There are, of course, multiple ways of dealing with these tests, and they must fit the personality of the woman chief. One response is to avoid confrontation, yet leave absolutely no doubt about who is in charge and who makes the decisions. Make it clear, however, that constructive suggestions are appreciated. The deputy of the preceding chief (who most typically was a man), may tend to gossip and often will try to make it appear that he is the one, running the show. Although this behavior might be tolerated for a short time, eventually she should call him in for a discussion of his responsibilities. The limits of his authority should be spelled out clearly, as uncertainty creates confusion and conflicts. It is totally up to the chief when and how to conduct such a meeting, depending on what she is comfortable with.

This brings back the well-known truism: A male executive can afford to be as aggressive as he wishes. And as long as he is predictable, even though unliked, he is endearingly referred to as "our son—of-a bitch." A woman executive, even if less aggressive, is just accorded the term of the canine female rather than the endearing term of the adopted offspring. In meetings she must give the impression of being cool, smart, deliberate, and in control.

The woman executive should also avoid touching. While men are allowed by consensus to "touch down" (to individuals of lesser rank than theirs), this behavior is not always welcomed from women. On the other hand, a cool buss on the cheek with equals or subordinates (only at levels close to yours) may be acceptable.

Making every word in public count is an art that must be learned, continuously perfected, and assiduously practiced. If in a meeting you feel that you are close to losing control (screaming or crying), look at your watch, and excuse yourself by saying that you have to leave because you are late for an important meeting. Remember, *Chiefs don't cry* (in public). Chiefs are cool, have a plan, and can handle any situation competently. It is still a man's world and women must play by the rules of the game but without surrendering their femininity. The same should apply to written correspondence and e-mail. While aides can write the letter for you, never allow an important letter or e-mail to go out without personally checking every word and considering its meaning. If its very important, postpone sending out the letter until the next day. Overnight reflection may provide you with a cooler head that will help you to omit emotional components to your message.

An interesting aside is that ambitious women at the same hierarchical level sometimes are jealous of each other, They may snipe and gossip.

They are, however, generally friendly and protective of their female aides and subordinates. Strong loyalties occur if the relationship has no competitive aspects. Men compete at a less personal level.

Women who are not upward bound often will bond with each other with greater ease than with men. While they easily can talk with other women about subjects of mutual interest, some women may not be interested in men's chatting about football, baseball or other sports. As painful as it might be, the woman executive may have to suffer through this type of conversation when among equals, even when this is an obvious attempt to differentiate her from her male colleagues. If, however, she is the leader, she should take control, change the topic, and divert the discussion to the business at hand.

In the man's traditional world (and increasingly in a woman's), many expressions are sports related, like "team player," "high scorer," "carrying the ball," "even playing field," to name just a few. Live with what you cannot change if it does not threaten your dignity.

In summary, to stay successful is to anticipate difficulties and have plans to deal with them. Have the vision and strength to look beyond the present and immediate future, and plan for at least five years ahead. Yet remain flexible and ready to alter tactics without losing sight of the ultimate goals. While these are general rules of leadership, women often surpass men in patience, attention to detail, strength, the instinct to anticipate difficulties, adherence to vision, and compassion. These unique qualities often are a surprise to their male associates.

STARTING:
THE DIFFERENT
APPROACHES AND THE
ENTRANCE SPEECH

Mix modesty and humility with the signals that you are sure of yourself and in control. Charm, wit, and dignity are a good combination. Ease out incompetents and replace them with ambitious, promising individuals. Don't have modest plans for the future: shoot for the stars.

Be aware that the arrival of a new chief is always threatening to the status quo. There will be rumors about your character, disposition, and style of running a show. Your previous record will be carefully scrutinized and every possible piece of gossip will be circulated and likely distorted through repetition. Remember that there is always an uneasiness about whether the new chief will bring a cohort of new people and the present staff will be slowly demoted or forced to retire or resign. The best way to avoid the divisiveness of "us versus them" is for the new chief to come alone, with only a raincoat over his or her arm. All the new people can then be chosen together with the existing staff, unless there is an urgent need for total revamping.

Before you start the new job, be aware that this is a new beginning, not only for you, but also for everybody in the enterprise. You can adopt a new style, select the manner of running the show, and portray the image that you wish to project for a long time. This means that you must be comfortable with that image and should not deviate from it, no matter what the pressures are. Being predictable is one of the important ways to prevent unrest and convey a sense of equilibrium. Being consistent does not impose any particular style of how you run the shop, it just limits how much you are allowed to deviate from the expected behavior. As you start, you should announce how you plan to proceed.

There are several scenarios for the first meeting with the whole staff. Probably the most propitious is to start with how happy you are to be appointed chief of this well-regarded (maybe even say "famous") institution. Compliment the quality of the staff and reputation of the entity. Even if everyone knows that the enterprise may have slipped, acknowledge that it is a "transient slippage" and assure the group that this can be remedied as the basic ingredients are in place or can be brought in. Say a few complimentary words about your predecessor and gauge the remarks according to his or her record (it would be inappropriate to praise excessively someone who has been fired for incompetence).

Be humble, even if your predecessor was a failure and you have been appointed to reverse a debacle. Be particularly self-effacing if he or she was an astounding success and you have to fill big shoes. Do, however, convey self-confidence. Do not single out for praise anyone else besides your predecessor. Those whom you mention by name will feel that they merit it and therefore you have not done them a favor. Those whom you omit will have been listening carefully to hear their name, and not hearing it, will be hurt, will remember, and will not forgive. Do not talk about plans

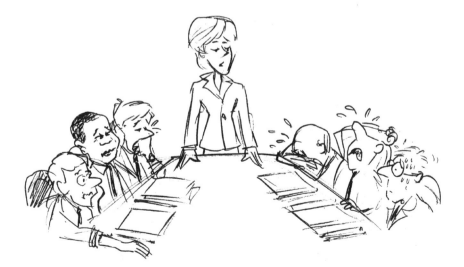

Any Questions, Gentlemen?

that may threaten the whole group. You may create a revolt before you have even started.

There have been instances where the new chief announced that previous commitments will not be honored, that important personnel changes will be made, and that the poor quality of the unit's performance will be reversed even if blood has to flow through the corridors. In at least one incident, this announcement alarmed the staff so much that, united by fear, they were able to get the new chief fired before he even had the time to assume the position.

Another new chief addressing the faculty in his new department told them frankly that he takes inspiration from Sun-Tzu's *The Art of War* and therefore his message to his staff was: "Follow me blindly, or I shall destroy you mercilessly!" This may be an excellent way to instill fear, but it is hardly an approach to gaining enthusiastic support!

As for keeping your predecessor's cabinet there are two approaches. The first is to start totally anew and dismiss them all. This is recommended only if you are in possession of enough information about the members and the entity you are starting to head, and you have an idea that in a relatively short time you will choose new confidants and a new cabinet. Although many new chiefs may find this approach attractive, it has disadvantages:

1. You are creating enemies unnecessarily.
2. Some dismissed members could be very helpful, as they have specific knowledge that may be invaluable.
3. Why hurry?

Another, much preferable approach is to keep the cabinet, add new members, and slowly start to replace the unwanted members, who are either not loyal or do not fit into your plans. Be careful and think carefully about the replacements. The dismissed individuals will be resentful unless you apply the Peter principle recommendation of creating a "lateral arabesque," inventing high-sounding, empty titles and jobs, such as "director of planning for future expansion." Saving face costs you nothing and avoids widespread ill will. The individuals that you keep will not necessarily feel more loyal when they realize that you have kept them because you need them.

In any event, first meet individually with each member of the cabinet of the previous head and get as much information as possible. Even if these initial meetings are unstructured, other meetings can be arranged later. Do speak with the incumbent chief. He or she may give you valuable information that is not public.

This is the time that you will remember the often quoted anecdote of the three letters: A new head of the department is meeting the outgoing head who gives him three letters with instructions to open them only one at a time, as numbered, and then only if in deep trouble. Soon after the beginning of the new regime, the subordinates are about to revolt, as their salaries have not been raised in five years and inflation is rampant. As the new chief believes that his job is on the line, he opens the first letter that says, "Blame the troubles on the bureaucracy and the previous adminis-tration." He does so and although things are not getting better, the revolt peters out. There is very little turmoil for a year or two, and then everyone in the institution is again up in arms and demands the chief's head. He eagerly goes to the second letter, opens it and finds the instructions, "Promise an urgent and thorough study of the difficulties, appoint a select committee, and swear to follow its recommendations to the letter." With these promises, the rational members of the revolt persuade everyone to be patient and a truce is called. As nothing improves, after a few more years, the rebels are again angrily confronting the chief. He eagerly runs to the third letter, opens it, and reads, "Prepare three letters for your successor!"

You may not look forward to accepting the three letters, but at least the first two may be helpful. While whatever you learn from your predecessor will probably be heavily biased and probably self-serving, it is rough data that properly sorted might be invaluable. If there have been several predecessors in a relatively short time, try to contact each one of them, and, if possible, arrange a social occasion including spouses. This approach is respectful, relaxes the atmosphere, and may facilitate the flow of valuable information.

It is a good idea to have a concept from the very beginning about where you wish to lead the institution. Examine whether expansion or shrinkage is required in order to make it better. You may need to diversify, invest a higher percentage of income into research and develop-ment, save resources, or invest everything in promising new directions. Even if you have good preliminary data, do not announce your plans unless you have restudied them once in the job, discussed them with trusted associates, and cleared them with superiors who could veto, delay, or mutilate them. Take several months to study everything: meticulously. Consider the quality of personnel in every area and at every level. Include space, equipment, and relations with other related entities within the mother institution as well as the outside world. Assess the physical ambience. Changes of furniture, decor, carpets, and so on may elevate the mood and signal that you care. It is advisable to meet with individual staff members. Meet with the most senior and select junior members individually. In one—on-one meetings you will learn more, and the privacy of the approach will be appreciated. Although this effort consumes a great deal of time, it is a very good investment.

THE FIRST MEETING WITH INDIVIDUAL STAFF MEMBERS

Mix modesty and humility, yet transmit the impression that you are sure of yourself, are energetic, have imaginative plans, and that you are in control. Listen! Convey that you are intensely interested in the well-being of each individual. These must be your true feelings. Sincerity has a way of coming through, while duplicity is difficult to dissimulate. Mix dignity with charm and wit, and show that you can be totally relaxed in any stressful situation.

The size and location of offices are critical factors as they convey rank and importance in the perception of the staff. Try to dispel that notion. Keep for yourself an office in a location that does not have the best view, is not overwhelming, and is located such that it does signal that you are the chief. The office should be well furnished with taste and touches of elegance but not lavish. It should be of medium size and comfortable for interviews. Remember that you are, from the beginning, establishing your style for the unit. Your associates will imitate that style to signal their importance and position on the totem pole.

After you have started, do not immediately make any major decisions regarding personnel, such as redistributing space between sections or divisions or abolishing or creating any new sub units. Use this period of study to meet with all subchiefs. Ascertain their impressions about the entity, as well as their plans and hopes for the future. Attempt to get them to feel relaxed and willing to open up and confide. Make frequent unannounced visits to the place where the work is done. Chat extemporaneously. Your presence indicates interest and a willingness to learn. Visit your equals to learn about their opinions about the quality of the entity you have just taken over as well as their plans for cooperation, use of your services, and willingness to be helpful.

After you have studied the situation, evaluated the members of your cabinet and leading members of the staff, and weighed their performances against your plans and expectations, there are two possible approaches you can take. One is to wait patiently and unobtrusively, affecting changes by having a few select individuals quit. This may take time, but it is nontraumatic and will generally, unless there is a crisis, lead to success. It does not create fear and if the people who are let go are found different face-saving positions elsewhere or are given, as stated before, "lateral arabesque" positions, you may create friends instead of enemies. Your message is nevertheless conveyed when ambitious, upward-bound, hard-working individuals replace incompetent personnel. Good taste is essential in the manner by which staffing changes are made.

Another approach, frequently used by some (but not recommended by me) is to find out who is the most unpopular of your potential opponents, and publicly dismiss him or her. This will convey the message that you are tough and powerful, and it will instill the proper respect and even fear in any potential troublemakers. Fear, according to this approach, is desirable, but hatred must be carefully avoided. Hatred is earned by attacking what is most precious to the "nobles"—namely, "possessions and honor" (Machiavelli in *The Prince*). This approach may backfire, particularly if not enough research has preceded the punitive action. The deposed "duke" may not have been as unpopular as you had estimated and may have influential friends Instead of making the staff become cooperative, you may have generated the beginning of a revolt. Obviously, this risky approach has many drawbacks, besides the fact that most present-day chiefs do not feel comfortable appearing overly tough. And in the United States, such a strategy may cause consternation in the personnel and legal departments of the institution (particularly the latter). Lawsuits against you and the institution are likely. The approach may work well in the armed services. In civilian life, however, although it may be successful, it does convey a clear style at the start of your tenure of being brutal, formal and distant. Unless the chief brings along one of his or her own top aides, there will be little intimacy between the chief and the top associates for a long time.

How does all of this apply specifically if the new chief is a woman? Although there may be individual differences, as shown by Indira Gandhi, Golda Meyer, or Margaret Thatcher, most women prefer the softer approaches described earlier. Generally they will choose to keep the inherited cabinet in the beginning and hope for help and loyalty from its members. The women chiefs will and should in their first address give praise to the staff and be perceived as warm, competent, enthusiastic, and fair. Toughness and harshness in a new woman chief does not evoke the same reaction as when the new chief is a man. In a man, these traits may be considered as acceptable, although not likable. In a woman, toughness and harshness are often considered unexpected, unusual, and threatening. A woman chief is generally expected to be warm and motherly.

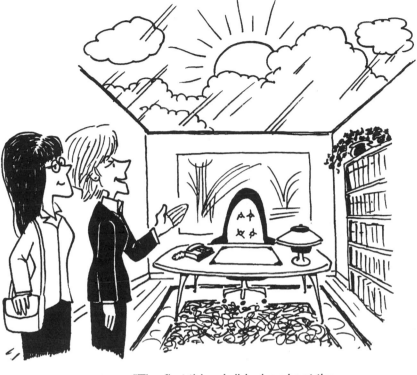

"The first thing I did when I got the president's office was install a glass ceiling."

As for early contacts with other members of the staff, the same behavior applies as for the male colleagues. Be friendly, dignified, and somewhat distant. Establish your own style. When choosing furniture, carpets, and art for the office suites, as a new chief generally does when starting, do not allow your feminine taste to be imposed on the whole group. Have a committee advise you. Otherwise the same rules apply. Do not be lavish in equipping your office and surrounding suite. Your selections may be even more carefully scrutinized than those of your male counterparts.

All new chiefs, however, should follow the basic rule of starting: After you have gotten your bearings and learned from the staff and colleagues about the anatomy and function of your domain, decide what you wish to accomplish. If you wish to leave a mark, try to shoot for the stars. Those who aim for modest, easily achievable goals will not engender enthusiasm and may not even reach the limited goals they have chosen.

THE DIFFERENCES BETWEEN ACADEMIC AND BUSINESS CHIEFS

The basic rules for survival and success are similar, the pressures are greater, and life is more difficult in business than in academia. The essence in both revolves around innovative ideas, people, space, and money.

I n the opinion of many who are not familiar with the differences between the military, academia, and business, a chief is a chief regardless of the organization. This could not be farther from the truth.

Because a discussion about military chiefs is beyond the scope of this book, and because the armed services rules are very complicated and totally different from those of business or academia, we do not deal with the subject of guiding a military chief's behavior. That type of a leadership manual would have to make the distinction between rules that apply to chiefs in peace and those in war. In the latter, the distinction between success and failure is much simpler. (The author's experience is limited to a two-year service as a medical officer, very far removed from the opportunity to observe the mores that military chiefs must abide by.) Therefore, this chapter will deal only with differences in rules that guide the careers of academic and business chiefs.

ACADEMIA

In discussing leadership in academia, I shall attempt to describe how the chiefs in the medical establishment, the law, engineering, and science, as well as art and humanities schools exercise leadership. In medical academia, there is a difference between what is expected from chiefs of clinical departments and what is expected of chiefs of basic science departments. To begin with, the exercise of the chief's power throughout academia differs only in form and ritual from what happens in the business world. The basics, when the cover of forms and tradition is lifted, are not that different. In all areas, the chief is supposed to make the department, school, campus, or business, grow in importance, space, equipment, number of satisfied customers, and income. The chief must provide opportunities for advancement and recognition for members of the department, school, or company. The yardstick by which success is ultimately measured differs. In business, achievement is measured by the value of the stock in established companies. In startup companies, it is the ability to raise investment funds for the expansion and fulfillment of plans, the closeness to becoming profitable, and the need to launch a high value initial public offering (IPO). In academia, the yardstick is more complex than the price of stock and profitability projections. It consists of total grant support, the number of times articles are quoted in the literature and the prestige of the journals, and the number of faculty members in the National Academy of Sciences and its branches, the Academy of Engineering, or the Institute of Medicine. Having Nobel laureates as faculty members is limited to only a few leading academic institutions, but this represents the ultimate in academic success.

For such achievements in academia, the chief must be able to provide adequate funds for the entity. This is so whether it is accomplished by fund raising, obtaining grants, or running the institution as a high-minded, civic-oriented, positive-balance business.

The differences in how clinical academic and basic science chiefs function are only superficial. Both control space, income, and promotions to higher academic titles. Titles are somewhat but not totally related to income. In the clinical departments of medical schools, the assignment of clinical duties is customarily the prerogative of the chief, and generally these decisions are related to income and prestige. (Consider Machiavellis *The Prince*—"possessions and honor"). The chief in clinical departments distributes the income earned by the practicing clinicians according to rules that must be carefully designed and approved by the school and university. The faculty members who earn it may not be invited to provide input. The size of the total clinical income depends on the hospital's outpatient facilities and the faculty's reputation in the community and country (in some teaching hospitals, reputation may also depend on international recognition). At each level of the academic hierarchy that allows the practice to prosper, taxes are imposed that support other necessary activities. These taxes start in the department, but the school, hospital, and campus collect them also. In state universities, a portion of the taxes also have to be returned to the state treasury. How does a clinical chief of an academic department succeed? The basic rules are the following:

1. Although you are chief of a department, you must balance the obligations to your department with service to the higher entity. Remember, when the ship sinks, the first-class sinks to the bottom too.
2. Your department is expected to deliver clinical care at the highest level, surpassing the care of community practices, yet because you are a teaching center, you are less efficient and costlier than the competition.
3. You must provide an environment that is encouraging and that facilitates research and innovation. This means that the faculty must be assured of research time. Some members of the department will either have fewer clinical duties in order to engage in research or will collaborate with basic scientists who guide the research. These part-time clinicians are expected eventually to be grant supported.
4. If you are dividing income among department members, you must apply an accepted formula in order to avoid the impression of favoritism or capriciousness. (This also applies to business entities, whether small or global.)
5. If you are a clinical chief, you should participate as a role model in earning the department's income, as this boosts morale. If the chief does not generate clinical income, the subchiefs will do as little as possible and this approach will be imitated all the way down the totem pole.

Heads of basic science departments and directors of research institutes in universities are similar to clinical chiefs only in the basic exercises of duties. In the daily, routine functions of leadership, they are almost indistinguishable from their colleagues in engineering, law, and schools of humanities. They also control space, which is of vital importance everywhere. Promotions are also very important, as they are related to prestige, salaries, and access to outside consultantships. As the academic duties mostly involve teaching and research, which are traditionally related to areas of interest, most of the power of such a chief is in the assignment of financial resources, space, assistants, and allowing and even finding opportunities for consultation or participation in industry. The opportunities for outside income vary greatly from school to school, geographic locale, and type of expertise. Written rules, accepted by consent and tradition, prevent academic chiefs from being capricious in the distribution of goods and assignments. The rules for success, again, are not very different. To be a successful chief or director of a basic science or engineering unit, one must do the following:

1. Establish a distinguished or even preeminent record in the discipline.
2. Continue actively participating in the field, thus assuring leadership and serving as a positive role model. This adds to authority.
3. Be a mentor to promising beginners.
4. Be as supportive as possible to members of your unit by giving them opportunities to become successful, even famous. Go out of your way to assure their financial success and be generous. Never compete with them.
5. The more prominent the members of you academic unit are, the greater the name of the institution is. This also makes it easier to obtain resources for continuous ascendancy. All of these factors will contribute to increasing your prestige. Remember, the conductor of an orchestra of virtuosi is sure to also become a celebrity. The well-worn phrase "nothing succeeds like success" has merit.

The hierarchical steps of authority in universities are somewhat misleading. Although on paper a dean should have much more real power than a department chief, the power structure varies greatly from school to school. It has to do with the following factors:

1. Rules of controlling departmental as well as individual income, earnings, and taxation
2. Rules governing the distribution of funds from endowment
3. Access to external fund-raising
4. Distribution of space

While deans and sometimes chancellors may control the distribution of space, this in practice, generally, applies only to new space. Possession is usually a strong reason for retaining space, unless the dean or chancellor wishes to foment unrest. Changing the status quo of space is almost always perceived as an ominous threat. Although this is very difficult for most deans to stomach, their mixing into the existing rules guiding the earning of income, increasing taxes, or taking away space, which has been part of a department for decades, often results in unifying the faculty against the dean and starts revolts. This may explain why deans have a shorter average tenure than do department chairs.

Chancellors and university presidents generally reign longer than deans and if forced to resign before retirement, this is most often due to their mishandling of a scandal in which they are rarely personally involved. The rules about how to handle a scandal involving a university often are confusing. A chancellor or president who deals sternly with a scandal may be forced to resign just as frequently as one who deals with the scandal mildly and tries to explain it away. The mere existence of the scandal may be enough to end a president's or chancellor's tenure. Occupying the university president's office is by now a frequent way for the students to protest. The handling of this type of action can create trouble for university administration. The secret of avoiding significant damage to the administration is to end the siege quickly and peacefully with reasoning, meetings, and hope that the student body will become bored. The administration should try to avoid media attention.

There is a difference in the aftermath of a forced resignation of a department chief, a dean, and even a university president from that of a business CEO. The academic chiefs almost always are university professors with tenure related to their academic teaching title, not their administrative position. If an academic chief chooses or is forced to give up the administrative post, he or she usually returns to the teaching post. Most often this more is associated with a significant loss of income. The leader will frequently take a year's sabbatical leave in order to renew skills. There are no golden parachutes, no increased perks or fringe benefits.

The survival prescription for an academic dean is as follows:

1. Rock the boat only very gently.
2. Build consensus.
3. Learn about unrest among the subordinate chiefs before they unite into a strong group.
4. Create feelings of pride about belonging to a school of excellence.
5. If you cannot provide the resources demanded, appear genuinely sorry to be unable to do so, causing the applicant to feel placated and sorry for the dean who wished to be generous, but could not because of circumstances beyond his or her control.

What rules apply to an academic chief if she is a woman?

1. Do not be more aggressive than the culture of the institution.
2. Be friendly, dignified, and somewhat distant.

3. Whether you are warm or cold in your contacts with subordinates, depends totally on the style that you are comfortable with. Just remain consistent and predictable.

4. Be protective of all young associates, but especially of young women. This is important because they still are more vulnerable than men, and this will continue until the culture changes even more than it has in the past two decades. Note that even in some politically correct medical institutions, it is rare to see a female department chair.

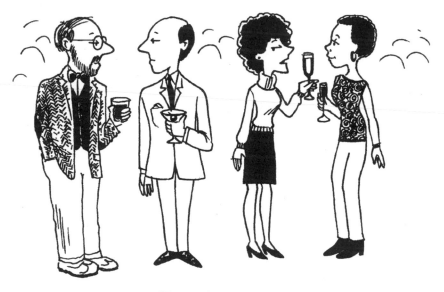

"Rumor has it they were separated at birth."

IN BUSINESS

The prescriptions for success for a chief in business are more complicated than for an academic chief. While all the basics are the same, the specifics differ. The rules vary according to whether the business is a startup, an established small business, or a large or even a global company. Some superficial rules even differ with the locale. While a chief of a startup in Silicon Valley is expected to be on a first-name basis with everyone in the company, this practice occasionally may be acceptable in the Midwest but is not universally practiced in the Northeast and the East Coast. The dress code for an executive of even an established (more than three years old) business in Silicon Valley and much of the West Coast is often but not always blue jeans, T-shirt, and sneakers. This would be unthinkable on the East Coast or in the Midwest.

STARTUPS

A startup chief should be the first among equals—visible, working harder than anyone to provide an example, friendly but stern, often a jack of all trades. The office in a startup is usually unpretentious, not much different than that of most of the associates. The chief's only security rests on the survival of the company until it is well funded and hopefully profitable. As the coworkers are paid poorly but work hard in order to make their stock options realize value, there is a general atmosphere of willingness to sacrifice for future gains. The morale of such a group is similar to that of a military unit engaged in combat. A successful chief encourages this atmosphere and is both a role model and morale builder. Such a chief has little security. The stock options over time may become valueless. Unless there is an unbreakable contract, the chief's stock options may disappear if he or she is fired or leaves the startup for greener pastures without the board's blessing.

As a very small proportion of startups survive the second or third drive for raising funds, the task of a startup CEO is formidable. Success generally depends on the timing, proper selection of associates, information, and vision that enables the CEO to choose the product and predict the demand for it. The CEO must anticipate ahead of the crowd what the public's trend and taste will be in the near future. Planning a startup for the distant future, no matter how bright, is a sure prescription for a short life for the company and the CEO's employment with it. Such a company should never be involved in manufacturing, at least not for a long time. Manufacturing requires a highly desirable product and a high demand for it. A great deal of expertise, experience, the assembly of an expert team, the timely purchase of building ingredients, and generally more funds than available are all essential for survival when manufacturing is involved. The mere assembly of associates experienced in manufacturing takes time and is expensive. Attempting it may spell the death sentence of the startup. The demise of a startup is often also due to the fact that even if the founder has a brilliant idea and is a great scientist, engineer, chemist, or computer whiz, he or she may have little knowledge about managing a business. The best combination is a Mr. Hewlett (engineering whiz) and Mr. Packard (a brilliant manager). With such a leadership combination, a startup in a garage became a global giant.

How do women perform in startup companies? Remarkably well. Perhaps this is due to the fact that those who succeed as CEOs are highly determined to prove that women can do it. But it is more likely that women who reach the top have vision, drive, and a powerful instinct for survival. Women that succeed as CEOs of startups generally display the following style:

1. They are friendly with associates.
2. They are able to generate the team spirit.
3. They recognize that bright young women seem to feel more comfortable placing their hopes for a successful career and future wealth with other women. Somehow they feel less likely to be exploited.

To remain successful, startups must grow, either by inventing new applications for their products or by developing new ones. Most important, whatever they do, they must improve continuously in order to stay ahead of the competition. To remain alive and be successful, the startup must grow rapidly, merge, or be profitably acquired by a large company.

SMALL COMPANIES

Chiefs of small companies must dream of transforming their businesses into large ones. They must reinvent themselves, grow with the innovations, and basically be similar to the startup CEOs (although they generally are not as stressed about being acutely short of funds). They also must show profit. There is no security for the chief, unless the business is family owned. Even then, if the business is faltering, a younger brother, sister, or an uncle may take over.

It is uncommon for a woman to head small company unless she is the founder. More frequently the woman leader is the favorite daughter or sister of the previous owner or, even more frequently, the surviving spouse. An interesting aside is that some women chiefs are more comfortable working with male associates than with women. The explanation— fewer jealousies and less jockeying for promotion. This is probably not common.

When small companies are not public, their chiefs enjoy sound sleep without the anxiety caused by fluctuating stock prices or quarterly reports.

Conversely, heads of small public companies generally have a life full of anxiety. Their length of service is similar to that of academic deans—short and eventful.

GLOBAL GIANTS

Numerous memoirs, biographies, and prescription books about leadership of giant, global companies might be summarized by the book *Only the Paranoid Survive* by Andrew Grove. This title may capture much of the essence for how a chief of a global company can stay successful and employed.

Unless the chief is a legendary, unique role model and icon like Jack Welch, the former CEO of General Electric, whose ideas and dictums in the business community rival those that Moses brought down from the Mount, the careers of global company CEOs can be similar to those of academic deans. Intrigues, mergers, double dealing, and treachery are sometimes seen on a large scale. *The New York Times Magazine* article on the career of Sanford Weill (with an unflattering portrait on the cover) reads like a textbook chapter on how to become a victim or a survivor in the top echelons of an evolving, hard-knuckle global giant.

This, however, does not have to be the rule. Heads of some giant, global companies have been selected by the boards for their inventiveness, previous successes, and demonstrated integrity. The basis of advancing such a giant company is to divide it logically into viable segments, appoint talented heads for each, give them freedom to grow without impinging on sister branches, and have them report and meet regularly in order to maintain cohesion.

For this style to succeed, the head of such a giant company must love his or her job and work long hours six to seven day weeks. He or she must carefully budget his or her time, have meetings start and end on time, and learn to listen in order to keep learning. The maxim "speak only if you can improve on silence" holds true no matter how high one's position.

HOW TO DRESS WHEN YOU
START

Clothes send a signal of beliefs and attitudes. Consistency as
well as inconsistency has its meaning.

M uch has been written about what to wear in academia as well as in
business, at the worksite, and for various social occasions. The
dictum that clothes make a career is a ludicrous exaggeration except in the
fashion industry. Clothes are more aptly the statement and expression of
the wearer's beliefs and desire to belong. In some ways, both in academia
and business, clothes at work are similar to uniforms in the armed
services: battle dress, station uniform, dress uniform, and so on. It is
said that the difference in wear between manual workers and executives is
that workers dress up at home and are in casuals at work, while the
opposite is true for executives. Executives dress well for work and most
try to look like bums at home, expressing their urge to relax.

The chief's dress code during his or her first few weeks at work will be
scrutinized closely by associates, particularly by women, as they tend to be
more observant in reading signals conveyed by clothes. A significant
deviation from what is expected makes an important statement at the
start one's tenure and, if repeated consistently, may establish a pattern to
be followed. The dress code is an important part of the first impression that
subordinates will gain upon seeing the chief during the beginning of
tenure. This is why it should be the object of careful planning. The options
should take into consideration several different standards, such as the
following:

1. Quiet elegance
2. Trendy, expensive, and showy,
3. Nondescript and easily forgotten (blending with the masses)
4. Sloppy

Each of these styles conveys a message more loudly than displaying a party membership card. Even neckties or scarves send signals. A Harvard or Yale tie or scarf, a Hermes, or a loud, multicolor Nicole Miller tie or scarf (preferably ill fitting with the suit or dress) can be interpreted easily as how the chief wants to be identified. Even apparently unimportant details, such as if the chief is seen with a Burberry raincoat or umbrella (or both) when entering or leaving the building, identify the chief's habits and preferences. Just remember, you should not be dressed like a model for designer wear one day and on the next appear as a customer of J.C. Penney's semiannual sale. Even this may not always hold. If you vary in wear widely from the most expensive Hermes, Kitan, Brioni, Versace, or such clothes to something obviously inexpensive and sloppy, initially you may confuse the imitators. But eventually the message will be understood: You can afford anything, but attire is unimportant to you and you are above it.

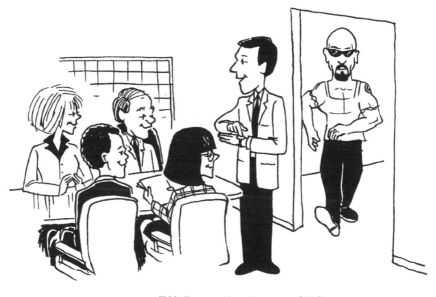

*"Well, people, the new CEO
should be here any minute."*

The head of a famous East Coast medical center wore black tie on appropriate official occasions and expensive suits and ties when meeting with the trustees, but enjoyed coming to the office in blue jeans, sport shirts, old windbreakers, and sneakers, while everyone else was obliged to don business suits and neckties. The message was clear from the beginning: The chief does not believe in the conventional, and he is above the rules.

HOW TO DRESS ONCE YOU
_____ ARE ESTABLISHED

As important as dress code may be, it is only part of the whole picture and should not be overestimated in importance. It is only one aspect of the total impression the chief will convey.

Once the pattern of dress is established, what is to follow? Obviously one must continue for the sake of consistency to dress in the general style you established during the first few months, whatever style you have chosen. A significant change from the first perception will be interpreted by the subordinates as a sign of lack of substance and potentially even as phony. Remember that your style will be imitated. Consistency and predictability are essential in dress, as is behavior, for a new chief. However, the opposite may be planned on occasion (see the previous chapter). Furthermore, as time passes gradual changes are almost expected, as everything changes with time, particularly fashion and style.

A chief in academia, especially one in business, is in many ways similar to a commanding general or admiral in that the dress code that he or she chooses may signal the message to conform. The dress code varies in civilian life much more than it does in the military, and the ways to make a statement through clothes are more numerous. Some forms have become almost traditional and obligatory for different groups, in academia as well as in business. For men, double-breasted dark suit with a fashionable silk tie on a clinical academic chief or the CEO of a business makes a statement about what he believes is proper in formal circumstances. This same outfit would cause derision in a basic science department where the message expressed by dress more typically includes a sweater, an open-collar shirt, blue jeans or corduroy pants, and any type of casual shoes. A sloppy, comfortable jacket is acceptable but not necessary to complete the picture. As stated previously, a business chief's dress may also vary according to the section of the country as well as the type of company. An example may be that some chiefs in academia and especially in business, may establish the Friday dress code as casual in order to evoke a mood of friendliness and togetherness. In some West Coast dot-coms, this may even mean shorts. For some parties and receptions, a certain type of wear that the chief recommends or even makes obligatory may become the expected dress code for associates.

Black tie for selected formal occasions is not uncommon in certain businesses and even at some academic events. White tie occasions are so exceptional in the United States that it does not merit a discussion here. Tails are worn by very few addicts to tradition and then only at some special state or social events such as the opening gala at the Metropolitan Opera, the San Francisco Opera, or some White House receptions when the president is *not* an egalitarian (an almost extinct breed).

Women chiefs have many more ways of expressing what they believe should be, the uniform for various occasions. For example, dark dress suits, suits with trousers, dark or multicolored bright dresses, if worn all the time at work, are an announcement of what the chief believes is proper for the unit, men and women. In academic and industrial basic science laboratories, and in certain parts of the country as in some industries, the dress code for women chiefs is totally casual, similar to that of their male colleagues. A statement is also made by the choice of corduroy pants, blue jeans, and running shoes or a loose, comfortable dress. Casual clothes also make a statement if they prominently display expensive designer labels. Being comfortable does not necessarily detract from elegance. Remember, walking with difficulty on high heels for the sake of appearing taller or more attractive may be perceived as a lack of good judgment. High heels that some women chiefs wear to work in order to appear more fashionable and elegant eventually take their toll. In some parts of the United States, particularly on the East Coast and in the South, women executives do not wear suits with pants at work, especially not in meetings with peers. Perhaps this is the result of a feeling among their male colleagues that women should not wear pants as it is not feminine, perhaps it is a subliminal expression of being uncomfortable with women ascending above the glass ceiling. The explanations are unclear, but the facts of this local custom are indisputable, yet slowly changing even there.

As important as the dress code may be, it is only part of the whole picture and should not be overestimated in significance. Again, it is only one aspect of the total impression that a leader will convey.

HOW TO USE YOUR OFFICE
AS A THEATER OF
OPERATIONS

Your office reflects a great deal about you and can be used to convey the message about how you wish to manage.

Your office is as important as your home and should reflect your personality, your beliefs, and the image you wish to project to your associates, your chiefs, and the rest of the world. The office location, size, furniture, decoration, flooring, carpeting, artwork, and diplomas (if any) are as revealing an expression as are your clothes (discussed in previous chapters). There is also an art to how to use the arrangements and furniture in the office to show that you are always in charge.

Your office should not have the best view. If there is a particularly symbolic monument, building, or view that would invoke patriotism or loyalty to the entity, it is smart to have the office oriented toward that symbol. Your associate should be seated so as to have an unobstructed view of it. This kind of positioning may change the atmosphere of a tense meeting.

Your office should not be larger than the norm for offices in your building, unless you wish to convey absolute power. Be careful not to be perceived as a vain megalomaniac. The best office location can be assigned to one of the midlevel associates. This demonstrates that you are modest, and it provides an additional benefit: As everyone knows that the best location has been assigned to someone who is not at the very top, location is deprived of importance, and you can avoid the pecking order that sometimes arises over office size and location. You should not carry this idea to the extreme, as did the late Dr. Julius Comroe, the legendary founder and director of the Cardiovascular Institute at the University of California, San Francisco. To combat the shortage of space and to curb the desire for large offices among his associates, he chose a cubicle for an office. Anyone not familiar with this symbolic gesture and who came to Dr. Comroe's office to ask for more personal space left without comment after seeing the size of his office. While this was an effective signal, it condemned Dr. Comroe to work in very restricted space. This is not recommended for claustrophobic chiefs.

It is important to understand that a chief is setting an example to be imitated. A large, elegant office incites competition, and imitation and it demonstrates the importance of rank. If space is limited, as it is in every successful operation (Parkinson's law), showing personal importance by having a large office is an unnecessary waste of resources. If the chief needs a site for small meetings (of 10 to 12 people at most) a conference room should be made available. It should be well furnished with some artwork, a beautiful table, a telephone that has a loudspeaker for telephone conferencing, and possibly video conference equipment. It is a mistake to have that conference room connected to the chief's office. It is better to give the message that conference rooms are a shared commodity, as space is precious. An example in point: The new head of a large department in a famous medical school that was notoriously short of space negotiated, at the time of his recruitment, to have a large, lavishly furnished office. As if this were not a sufficient blunder, he also had a conference room–library, which was of course, equally beautifully arranged and built with access only through his own office, as if to show that his reign was supreme (*L'état c'est* moi, as Louis XIV put it succinctly, leading to the end of Louis XVI). Needless to say, this chief committed other similar errors, was the object of ridicule, and had a very short tenure. The furniture and the total ambience of the office, wallpaper, statuary, floor, carpets, even diplomas should be thought out carefully. While it is advisable to have an interior decorator in order to save time and aggravation, take time to instruct her or him about your taste, the message your office is to emit, and the impression you wish to convey about how expensive it was to furnish.

The office reflects a great deal about you, and in many ways it can be used almost as a weapon. The desk expresses power as you sit behind it. The higher the back of your chair, the more it conveys the impression of high rank. I would advise you to have at least two armchairs, not extremely comfortable, in front of the desk. (In order to make meetings with people sitting in these chairs as brief as possible, one CEO of a large company had the seats of these chairs arranged at a downward slant. People could not wait to get up.) A table, as beautiful as your budget can afford, with four graceful chairs around it is a useful component of a functional executive office. A couch requires the office to be larger, but if feasible,

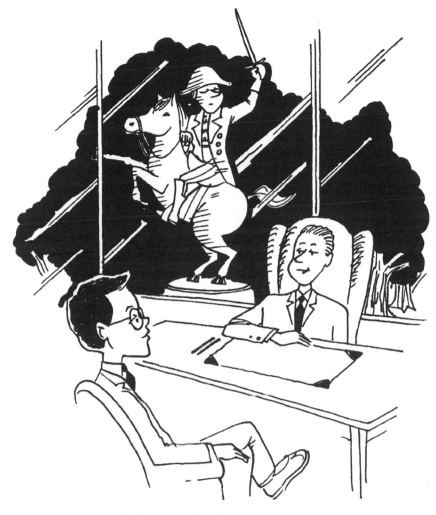

"Why, yes, that is me young man. ·
How astute of you to notice."

without crowding, it might allow for an afternoon nap (when no one is watching and if the administrative assistant can be trusted not to tell anyone that the chief is sleeping during working hours) (a short nap may be a godsend on stressful days).

How does one use the furniture to create the desired atmosphere in which the meeting is to take place? If the chief wishes to discipline one of the subordinates, he or she must sit behind the desk with the culprit sitting in a chair in front. This signals the distinction in positions. For praise or for a work session, the chief and the visitor (or visitors) can sit at the table in the office. If there is a couch, and you wish to be friendly, a male chief can have a male visitor or associate sit on the couch, or you may both sit on it. A male chief should never do that with a woman associate or visitor. She will generally feel very uncomfortable and the whole meeting may become tense and awkward. A woman chief will almost never have a couch in her office.

If space is not terribly limited (unfortunately, it generally is), a wonderful way of saving time and being efficient is for the top executive to have a second small office, known only to the trusted administrative assistant and very few chosen lieutenants. There, the chief can work free from unscheduled visitors who intrude and—although promising to finish their business in a few minutes—stay until it becomes embarrassingly clear to them that they are a nuisance. If the chief continues to engage in research or engineering work, this second office can be attached to a laboratory or workroom. However, it should never become a place for meetings, as its primary purpose as a retreat for unimpeded work is then jeopardized.

If the company or department has several locations, the chief may maintain offices in each, depending totally on the distance between them. Although there is nothing absolute about it, the rule of thumb should be the following: Separate offices in different components of the business or academic department should be maintained only if the distance between them requires staying overnight. However, if the company has planes or helicopters available for transporting executives, which is possible only in very rich corporations, the previously postulated time restrictions applicable to other mortals do not apply here.

HOW TO BUDGET
YOUR TIME

Time is your most precious commodity. There are many ingenious ways to save time and be more effective. Long hours are not a substitute for functionality.

The difference between effective executives and those who are less so essentially comes down to how well they use their time. When everything is analyzed, everyone from the most junior employee to the most exalted chief has only 24 hours in a day. If one subtracts time for sleeping (seven hours), eating three meals (average: two hours), personal care and unmentionable activities (one hour), commuting to and from work (one hour), watching news on television or reading a newspaper (one hour), activities of daily living including time with one's spouse and children (a wise investment), socializing, exercising (three hours), and entertainment or obligatory dinners with associates or business prospects, one is left with only 10 hours to dedicate to work and some leisure. Very few of us can work 10 hours day in and day out. As I have been rather stingy in allotting time for various daily activities, it becomes obvious that an effective chief is left with a limited amount of usable time. The task at hand then is to use the time wisely and plan ahead. Probably the most important concept in budgeting time is to know what is essential to fulfill your mission and have that time take precedence over all else.

There are few rules for using one's time efficiently:

1. Delegate routine chores that need no decision making to trusted associates.
2. Instruct your office staff to scan and eliminate junk mail and show you only what you need to see.
3. Have the staff filter phone calls and preview e-mail. (It is important to train the staff on what is important, to whom you must talk, and what

you must see. If staff members are ever in doubt, have them say that you will call the person back.) Insist on seeing all material that might be important. This may avoid headaches. People who decide what you must and what you do not have to see are your most trusted assistants.

4. Establish priorities and do not waste the time on unnecessary activities.

5. Have a daily schedule prepared, and preserve unscheduled time slots (preferably 10 percent of your appointment time). This gives you flexibility. (Note that not everyone who wishes to see you, should be seen by you. Perhaps your staff can refer such people to someone else.)

6. Have cabinet and all scheduled meetings start on time (it is amazing how much time is lost—yours and everyone's else's—by every meeting starting 15 minutes after the scheduled start time as principals drift in late).

7. Chair the meetings in your unit. This gives you the opportunity to start on time, interrupt unnecessary chatter, and conclude the meeting when your objectives have been met.

8. Larger staff meetings should not be held in your office. If you wish, you can leave and let your deputy continue.

9. Meetings in your office should not be scheduled to last beyond 30 minutes. They should be programmed about a topic. Brain-storming, free-wheeling meetings are a luxury that can be reserved for relaxed retreats. Have several clocks in your office so that you are always aware of what time it is and how long the meeting has lasted without looking demonstratively at your watch.

10. If certain members of your staff need to "touch flesh" and see you repeatedly and unnecessarily, have them schedule an appointment in three weeks, by which time the " urgent" reason for the meeting may have evaporated.

11. Inform your administrative assistant how long the meeting in your office is to last. A few minutes before that time, have your assistant telephone you to remind you that you are needed elsewhere. You may even have a prearranged signal to buzz your assistant, so that if the meeting could be cut short, she or he can then make the required call that ends the meeting. It is rude for the chief to end the meeting by standing up, unless this is planned as a punitive message.

The essential ingredient in all of these suggestions is to have highly competent office staff who know your habits, are loyal, do not gossip, and know your taste and values. This cannot be overemphasized. It takes delicate judgment to know when to give someone an immediate appointment and when to convince someone else that you wish you could see him or her but it is just not possible.

Discretion and tact are essential in stopping a meeting with a visitor in your office. One head of an academic department had an hourglass very prominently displayed in his office. As a visitor would sit down, the chief would demonstratively turn the hourglass over and tell the visitor that it is programmed to empty the top in 30 minutes, which is how long the meeting will last. The visitor would squirm, and during the whole meeting, the hourglass would be the center of attention. Needless to say, this dedication to efficiency did not make the chief popular.

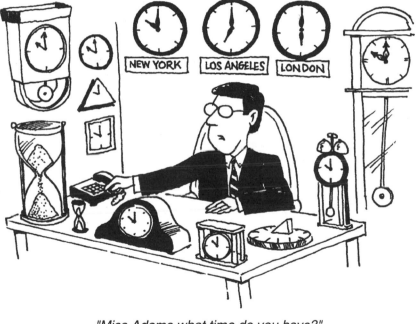

"Miss Adams what time do you have?"

There are other better ways of saving time. Realize that if a meeting with a subordinate is scheduled for 30 minutes, it might be considered rude to have the meeting be shorter. It may convey the message that the visitor is unimportant. Even getting up from the chair and thanking the visitor for coming, thus terminating the meeting, may be awkward. Being in the chief's office as long as possible is considered by many to be a matter of prestige. There are two ways of saving time while not being offensive and actually earning points:

1. Have your staff call the person who was supposed to come to your office and inform him or her that you will be there nearby and will come to his or her office. You score doubly because (a) you have shown respect by coming to the associate's office yourself, and (b) as you are the visitor, you can get up at any time, after the matter for discussion has been concluded (which you can usually achieve within 10 minutes). After a few minutes of friendly chat, you can get up. You have not only saved 15 minutes, but you have also shown the associate that you are friendly and respectful. By visiting the associate's office, you are also obtaining additional information about the associate's personality and tastes.

2. Have your administrative assistant give you the day's schedule. At least one or two hours before a scheduled meeting in your office, arrange to walk by the office or workplace of the person with whom you are scheduled to meet. Say that you were passing by and noticed on your schedule that you were to meet later. Ask if it would be convenient to discuss the matter of interest now, even if in the corridor. The usual answer is "yes, of course." The meeting then lasts only 10 minutes at the most (standing in corridors is not nearly as comfortable as sitting in the chief's office). You have saved 20 minutes and in addition you have shown how informal you are. There is a third advantage. By walking through the department or business, you are seen, you greet people who work for you, and you show interest in them. Furthermore, you may even learn firsthand about the operation by seeing people at work. David Packard, the cofounder of Hewlett-Packard, practiced "managing by walking through."

Do not work yourself into ineffectiveness. Very long hours may result in wasting time. Furthermore, some people are at their best in the evening, others in the morning, according to each individual's own circadian clock. Try to adjust your working hours to your inner clock. Efficiency can save time and improve the quality of the product. Realize that long hours are not a substitute for functionality. Do not run from meeting to meeting. Allow yourself time to think. Remember also that things not worth doing are not worth doing well.

GAINING RESPECT

You gain respect by being consistent, honest, courageous, and a positive role model. Do not ask anyone to do what you are not prepared to do yourself.

Being respected by superiors, associates, and subordinates should be the goal of every chief. Respect from associates and subordinates is the highest achievement to which an executive can strive, as it means that the people who are directly in contact with him or her have arrived at this judgment on their own, not by reputation. It is obvious that respect must be earned, and that it requires more than one or two actions. Consistent demeanor and actions over a long period of time earn respect. Respect is not easily gained. This is particularly true when it comes to gaining the respect of subordinates. It is only natural for everyone to look at a new chief with a mixture of doubts and high expectations about good predictions that have preceded his or her arrival.

Gaining respect has nothing to do with the mode of running the show. A chief can be stern, authoritarian, hard-nosed or friendly, easily accessible or warm, insipid, subdued, or colorless. Yet none of these modes of behavior will cause a chief to gain or lose respect. It is the attributes of personal honesty, dedication to justice, fairness, and consistency in treatment of all subordinates according to accomplishments and achievements that bring respect. Treating individuals with consideration, regardless of rank or connections, rejecting favoritism, serving as a role model by working hard and taking on difficult tasks is a sure way of gaining respect. Financial transparency and absolute honesty are essential.

Although this book addresses leadership in academia and business, it is the example of how leaders in the armed forces gain respect that can be a guide for all heads of functioning units to follow. In the armed forces, leadership is of paramount importance, and the results of poor command at high levels can be immediate and disastrous. Hence, some of the basic rules of military leadership are universally applicable. Abiding by these rules does not imply that the leader is being militaristic or preparing for warfare. However, as subordinates who follow a military leader may risk everything dear to them, including their lives, they will not do so voluntarily and with enthusiasm if they lack respect for their leader.

These rules, though simple, are not easy to follow as they may clash with the enjoyment of power, its perquisites, and the feelings of self-importance that inebriate many a chief. Here are some of these important guidelines:

1. Have no favorites. Everyone in your unit is your responsibility and is to be treated equally and fairly.

2. Do not demand anyone in your unit to suffer hardships that you are not willing to undergo yourself.

3. Be the last in the "chow line" (where perquisites or rewards are given) and first in the firing line (where hard work and perils are joined).

4. Be modest and inspire by example.

5. When you delegate, encourage success yet do not try to share the credit. Be generous and acknowledge the efforts of others.

6. Be charitable with those who fail. Do not destroy them, but find them assignments in which they will succeed.

7. Be able to make decisions that are hard on others, but do not make them without careful consideration.

8. Praise and distribute honors in public. Chastise, correct, and punish in private, unless you perceive that it must be done publicly in order to raise morale.

9. Select your style of command and do not deviate from it.

10. Never show doubt, even if you feel it. Confidence is as infectious as are fear and uncertainty.

11. Control your emotions and always appear cool in public.

12. Never reveal your thoughts.

13. Even when you raise your voice in anger, do it on purpose. If you cannot control a display of temper or strong emotions in public, excuse yourself and leave.

14. If you have to chastise an associate, do it in private and be as mild yet as precise as you can in describing the associate's error. This is a way for the guilty person to blame only himself or herself. Harsh criticism will often evoke the response "perhaps I made a mistake, but the boss had no right to be so harsh with me."

15. The system of remuneration must be uniform, logical, with built-in bonuses for high performance and hazards.

How do women chiefs gain respect? Is there a difference? There apparently is in our male-dominated society. Professor Higgins's lament in *My Fair Lady*, "Why can't a woman be like a man?" remains a widely held concept. It is due to that perception (prejudice) that for women to be successful they must behave like men. Women chiefs are more critically scrutinized than their male counterparts, almost in order to establish whether they behave differently than men. Women chiefs are aware of it and generally try harder, which can result in tenseness, longer hours at work, and some insecurity. Some try to cover this insecurity by being more harsh and harder on their associates and subordinates than are most men. Some, when they achieve the ultimate in the department's structure and power, start wars rather than pursue peace in order to show how tough they are. There are numerous examples of this type of behavior.

While it may be easier for a woman to reach the top today compared with the prior generation, this move up is generally based on superb performance at a lower level. Exercising leadership, however, may be less comfortable and more frightening to a woman once she pierces the glass ceiling and achieves the position of chief.

So how does a woman stay on top, be successful, keep her peace of mind, gain and retain respect? She should follow the same basic rules of leadership as men, but not change the natural behavior that brought her to the top. There is no need to impress and convert the doubters and male chauvinists by changing one's demeanor. Consistent behavior, reliance on facts, natural behavior, avoidance of exaggeration in dress, speech, or body language will reassure and even endear the doubters. Even if it is true that women tend to be, generally, but not universally, more emotional than men, this if controlled, can work as an asset. Show that you really care about important issues, that you are willing to risk much to achieve what you believe is right, and express yourself with feeling. This will engender more respect than many men will ever enjoy. The rectitude, warmth, and devotion to the welfare of those entrusted to the woman executive, particularly to those in trouble, stimulates the instinctive regard that one has for one's mother. This should not be considered as a weakness, but as a strong positive attribute. However, it cannot be overemphasized that even strong emotions should not lead to tears and sobbing in public unless this display of emotion is carefully planned for the appropriate effect. Chiefs don't cry (unless they plan to).

GAINING LOYALTY

Loyalty goes beyond respect. It is given after the chief demonstrates repeatedly that everyone's well-being, as well as that of the enterprise he or she heads, is of paramount importance. The Ten Commandments for gaining loyalty follow.

Loyalty to the chief goes beyond respect. Respect can be attained without associates or subordinates being willing to go through flood or fire for their chief. To gain this type of devotion from one's followers, the chief has to prove to be willing to reciprocate by doing the utmost for the welfare of those entrusted to him or her. Caring must be genuine, as pretending is easily detected, and it will make the leader lose face. It may even breed enmity. Loyalty too, is not gained overnight, but has to be acquired through repeated trials.

Although associates and subordinates are generally all adults, they often exhibit the feeling that "their" chief should behave like a parent who is supposed to take care of difficulties, make sure that everyone has secure employment, recognize hard work, and reveal "gold bricks" (people who pretend to be working) as such. The chief must be available to listen to reported problems and always have the right answers to one's troubles. Having an "open door," listening, sometimes being stern, always being interested and compassionate is the expected behavior of a good chief. The chief should not disclose doubts, reveal sleepless nights, or demonstrate worry about the future. Associates (like children) do not wish to share the burdens of leadership. They want the chief to take case of important decisions that assure their survival and well-being, as that is why he or she has been appointed (generally not elected). This type of relationship can be compared to that of the crew to the skipper of a ship. Everyone does his assigned duty, but the captain decides what is best for the ship. As long as the captain is judicious, maintains discipline, cares for the welfare of the ship and the crew, succeeds in whatever tests the ship encounters, and assures that everyone is safe and that sacrifices are appreciated and rewarded, the captain eventually will gain the crew's loyalty.

It is important and cannot be stressed enough that praise must be public and justified in the eyes of the equals to those who receive it. Public criticism should be reserved only for egregious mistakes that endanger the enterprise. Even then, the criticism must be handled fairly and not in anger. Should the chief make a serious mistake that requires disclosure, it is important that he or she acknowledges it and accepts responsibility. By disclosing the mistake to associates and never blaming anyone else, the chief shows that he or she deserves the backing and loyalty of those associates. This support will permit the unit to sail through any storm, because the group is standing by its chief. Top executives often believe that loyalty from subordinates at lower levels is automatic (if needed at all), because of the great difference in rank. To the contrary, not only does the chief need the loyalty of the highest-ranking associates for the success of the operation (and for the chief to keep his or her job), but he or she should *earn* everyone's loyalty. All on board must do what is expected in order for the enterprise to succeed.

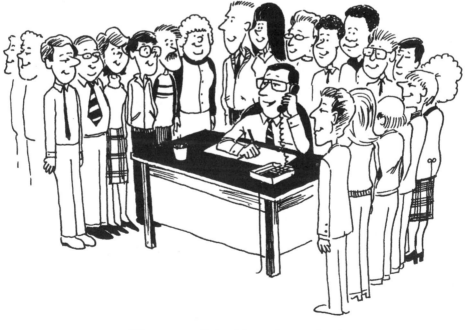

"Everyone pitched in and we solved
the office shortage problem."

It is only appropriate here to tell a story that exemplifies to an extreme the need to earn loyalty. It concerns a navy captain who had a brilliant career during one of the world wars, was slated for many promotions, and was expected to go to the very top. However, he had one major fault: He took full credit for any success of his ship but was merciless to people committing the smallest error. His ship was very visible, was the pride of the navy, and was in some ways the symbol of national victories. Returning from a glorious tour of ports in which the ship was feted, it ignominiously got stuck on mudflats not too far from its home port. As was customary in that country's navy, a board of inquiry found the captain blameless, but he was retired soon afterward, at a relatively young age, without being promoted. The true teaching impact is revealed by the fact that when the ship went on the mudflats, a full complement of naval officers was on the bridge along with the captain. It turns out that he was the only man on the bridge who was ignorant of the fact that the ship was headed at full speed straight toward the mudflats. The officers on the bridge knew that the captain ultimately would be held responsible and would be blamed for the shameful incident. This was the way for the crew to get even. The lesson to be learned by every chief is the following: If you wish to avoid having your ship get stuck on mudflats, earn the loyalty of your staff by giving credit to those who deserve it and assuming responsibility for mistakes.

Can a stern, tyrannical chief earn the loyalty of his or her staff? The answer is yes. The style of leading is not as important as the consistency, the caring, and the willingness to go all out for the welfare of the enterprise and the "crew." As long as staff members feel that the chief has everyone's interest as a matter of priority, and not only his or her own, the style of behavior is accepted even though it may be considered harsh.

The basic ten commandments for receiving loyal support from staff then are the following:

1. Be approachable.
2. Treat the staff with equal respect regardless of rank.
3. Care about individual problems of the people working for you.
4. Recognize success and reward it.
5. Distribute credit lavishly yet judiciously.
6. Be modest about your own accomplishments.
7. Convey a feeling of order and justice.
8. Do not disclose insecurity about the future.
9. Exude confidence.
10. Freely show the only emotion to be displayed—enthusiasm.

Carl Sandburg relates an interesting story about President Abraham Lincoln. Apparently Lincoln's secretary-receptionist was fastidious about giving appointments. President Lincoln took great pleasure in bringing visitors and associates whom he liked into his office by way of a side door, without appointments, thus bypassing his secretary. Thus, the president gained both respect and loyalty.

Must a woman chief behave differently to earn loyalty? It may be easier for her to obtain it from female employees, as instinctively they may feel that they are in the same boat. It may be more difficult for her to gain loyalty from male employees, however, particularly if they were there before the woman chief was put in the position of authority. Again, two principal approaches apply:

1. You may behave with sternness. Apply the Ten Commandments enunciated earlier with fairness but detachment, making sure that you are consistent.

2. Or you may apply the Ten Commandments in a manner that is both loving and warm, going out of your way to make people who work for you feel valued and cared for.

While we have emphasized the importance of caring and compassionate behavior on the part of the chief one cannot overstate how important it is for the chief to be (in addition to all of the above) competent, able, and successful in order to gain loyalty as well as respect. Compassion for a failed chief has a place only on visits to the hospital or funerals.

HOW TO TREAT CLOSE
ASSOCIATES

Close associates are most important in determining how a unit functions. Harmony and performing together as a smooth-functioning machine are essential for the success of the enterprise. Choose the members carefully, inspire them, listen to them, but be their leader.

M any experts on management and efficiency have said that clear and timely communication is indispensable for the success of any organization. This is even more important when operating with close associates. Always keep communications open with them. Simply assuming that they remember what was agreed upon or, even worse, making assumptions about what they should expect will inexorably lead to confusion and unhappiness. Close associates to the chief are often insecure, jealous, and even paranoid. This is particularly true during transitions.

Remembering the following basic rules on how to treat your close associates is essential:

1. Communicate clearly and continuously. Remember that what may appear unimportant to you but involves an associate's area of responsibility becomes vital to that person's ego. If associates find out that you have acted unilaterally, you may have created enemies.
2. Never get involved in power games by pitting one close associate against another.
3. Choose close associates according to the following precepts: for their (a) diligence, (b) proven accuracy and timeliness in providing data, (c) Efficacy in running their respective sections, so that you can delegate and have no surprises on review, (d) ability to handle personnel assigned to them, (e) loyalty to the greater unit, (f) ability to fit in as team members, and (g) ambition, which they exercise without being devious

or disloyal. Most of these attributes become obvious once you review each prospective close associate's previous record. Remember that the previous record predicts future performance. Few adults change their basic traits and behavior. As delegation of responsibility makes you effective, make sure that the individuals can perform the delegated duties

4. Treat your associates with respect. Judge them fairly in evaluations. Although they may be your age or even older, because they depend on you, your manner of treating them must be that of a loving parent or a protective older brother or sister. Tact is essential and you should go out of your way to be tactful. Always ask your close associates for advice, and show respect for their contributions and expertise.

5. Before criticizing and expressing unhappiness with an associate's actions, try an important mental exercise. Imagine yourself in the reverse role: If you were the associate on the other side of the desk, how would you like the leader to convey the bad news to you? If you come to the conclusion that you would like to hear it brought to you tactfully, with suggestions for improvement and with the clear message that the chief is here to help you and not destroy your career, the manner for disciplining your associates becomes easy and clear.

6. Discuss future actions. In difficult times you may find out that your close associates may be uniting against you. Face them openly. Convince them that in crises the team spirit is essential for survival. Instill the feeling that you are all one unit, a close-knit team: "One for all and all for one." This mode of behavior will carry you through many storms.

7. Close associates must be assigned well-defined duties. Preventing them from infringing on each other's territory avoids turmoil. Information about the goals, expectations, and methods must be disseminated and discussed. Decisions should be arrived at jointly and expected to be followed.

8. Do not dominate your team so vigorously that the decisions arrived at are basically yours, because your associates did not dare to antagonize you.

9. Avoid creating an undisputed second-in-command who may not be loyal. Having two such people, as suggested by the Peter principle, with a clear division of responsibilities, is a better way of keeping the unit on course. These two can alternate substituting for you when you are away. Remember, with cellular phones and e-mail you are never too far away. An outstanding individual, close to retirement, for example, may be acceptable for a single second-in-command. That

person may wish to retire in a blaze of achievement, thus demonstrating your good judgment in the selection (Vice President Cheney may be an excellent example of a loyal, most helpful and wise deputy).

10. Do not have favorites. Treat all your close associates equally, as if they were members of your family.

11. Unless you own the business privately, do not have members of your family (wife, sons, sons-in-law, daughters, daughters-in–law, nephews, etc.) as members of your inner council. Do not even employ members of your family in your unit. It is harder for them than for others to function and excel because nepotism is always suspected. If for some reason one of your family members has to be employed in your unit, you should not have any supervisory or controlling responsibilities for his or her performance.

A dramatic example illustrates this point: A very well known and highly respected head of a large unit in a prestigious, leading company employed a gifted, yet very undiplomatic son-in-law as a junior executive. The young man went out of his way to create enemies by openly criticizing and demeaning his peers. When he made a major mistake, everyone in the unit that had been hurt by his previous actions got together, and several of the chief's close associates demanded the son-in-law's immediate dismissal. The chief appointed a small board of inquiry to investigate matters. This group included close associates, yet the chief did not recuse himself from receiving report of the board. The board of inquiry reported to the Company's chairman of the board directly, thus bypassing the chief of the unit (the father-in-law) as well as the president and CEO (believed to be the chief's friend), and demanded the dismissal of both the father-in-law and the son-in-law. The case created national news and ugly rumors. All of this resulted in the chief's resignation, ending a distinguished business career. The son-in-law, young and talented, was immediately hired by a competing firm.

One important message that the chief must convey—without anger, coolly but emphatically—is that members of the inner circle do not talk ill about their chief if they wish to keep their position in the hierarchy. Suggestions and constructive criticism by cabinet members are welcomed, but only behind closed doors, privately, and directly to the chief one on one. Freedom of expression does not apply to speaking against policies that one was supposedly involved in designing.

When dealing with inherited close associates, the new chief should conduct the meetings in his or her own office in an atmosphere of friendly politeness that can, if needed, be turned into ice.

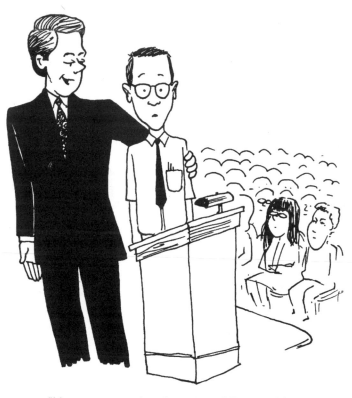

"Unaccustomed as I am to public speaking, I'm having Reynolds here read my speech."

A woman chief should handle her close associates in a like manner. If the associates are inherited from the previous regime, she should follow the rules enunciated in the chapter titled "Starting: The Different Approaches and the Entrance Speech." She need not tolerate being treated differently because she is a woman. If necessary to convince the inner council (the cabinet) of her determination, she should show the group her teeth. Still, it is usually better to be tolerant, to listen thoughtfully, and to remain dignified and firm. Rather than immediately altering the basic composition of the inner council, she can appoint new members solely on their worth. This rule should also apply to appointing other women. As with all effective chiefs, she should keep her close associates informed and be concise in communicating with them. All that was said above about gaining respect and loyalty applies doubly for women chiefs in dealing with close associates.

The close associates, who compose the inner council (the cabinet) are extremely important in determining how a unit functions. Harmony and performing as a smooth, functioning machine are essential ingredients for success. Therefore, the importance of choosing the members, inspiring them, and listening to them while still being their leader cannot be over-emphasized.

HOW TO TREAT EQUALS

Your equals can be the most important allies in battles. They will generally respond to collegiality, generosity, and your willingness to sacrifice your own unit's interests for the broader welfare of the company or university. Develop long-lasting friendships with them, and try to recreate Camelot.

Every university or business has a hierarchy in which the head of a branch, subsidiary, or department has equals. Your colleagues' units may be larger, smaller, or equal to yours in size or importance. This should be irrelevant to you. What is important is your state of mind in considering these people as your natural allies, helpers, and possible protectors rather than as competitors. It is important to do everything possible to avoid open disagreements in meetings with them. Try to train yourself to see only positives in your colleagues, and attempt to imitate those you respect the most. This attitude will unconsciously be expressed in your body language and generally will be met by a similar response from your colleagues. Equals usually respond in kind to friendly gestures. However, try to emphasize and follow a few basic rules:

1. During meetings with other chiefs in your company or university, leave your unit's hat at the door and don the cap of the larger entity.
2. Never be emotional in your contacts with your equals, unless you both (or all in larger meetings) share the emotion.
3. If you feel that you cannot control an outburst, excuse yourself and leave the meeting.
4. Do not preach. Speak only if you can improve on silence.
5. Back up all your statements with facts.

6. Never try to dominate a meeting with equals. If they are impressed with your leadership, knowledge, and behavior, your colleagues will back you.

7. Do not present important issues for your unit at a meeting before thoroughly preparing your material.

8. Be sure that your proposals are ultimately in the interest of the larger unit

9. Meet with the possible adversaries to your proposals before the presentation in order to avoid confrontations at the large meeting. Try to convert them.

10. Find powerful allies to your proposal and brief them thoroughly in advance.

11. While it is a bad idea to have personal or family friendships with close associates, subordinates, or whomever reports to you, close friendships with equals are to be encouraged. Such sincere friendships help you and the others to grow as leaders. They are beneficial to all sides, including the company or university, provided that you are not forming juntas for your personal interest and benefit.

12. Invite your friends who are your equals in the larger enterprise to your family celebrations.

13. Keep your equals informed about the plans for your unit even before presenting them to the common superiors. You should share what you have in mind with them.

14. The most common cause for dissension among equals is the distribution of funds and space. Remember that generosity, unselfishness, and cooperation are easy if your unit is rich and does not require funds, additional buildings, or more space. If your unit is rich, give generously and do not ask reciprocity in return.

15. If your unit is poor, you do not have the luxury of options that the rich have, so you must be inventive, innovative, creative and persuasive. Building from a poor base requires good leadership and, most of all friends in high places.

16. Never brag about your successes. This is the surest way to have your workplace friendships come to a quick end.

17. The friendships and warm contacts with your equals should endure even after each of you has retired. They contribute to making your careers worthwhile and provide a good example for your successors to follow, thus making peer friendships valuable to the company or university.

While these general rules of behavior will work in most instances, special situations may require different approaches. Do not get fixed in your approaches.

You may, for instance, have a colleague chief who is friendly on the surface, but is jealous of your successes and is trying to diminish them by taking every opportunity to undermine you and deprecate your achievements. This colleague may even obtain advantages, whether financial or in other ways (more office or work space, for instance) at your expense. It becomes a challenge, then, to determine how to best treat someone who is doing the total opposite of what a colleague should do when relating to equals. The surest way is as follows:

1. Remember that this colleague likely exhibits the same behavior to other equals and will eventually pay the penalties for it. So be patient and do not have confrontations.

2. Do not give in. Do not get emotional. Have facts about what the colleague is criticizing and strengthen your friendly relations with the rest of the group. Selfishness and lack of regard for the interests of the larger unit will eventually result in (a) lack of regard for the individual and (b) lack of power for the deviant. However, remember not to attribute to malice what can be attributed to incompetence.

How should a woman chief treat her equals in a university or company? While the rules are the same, if a woman chief is an exception rather than the norm for that company or university, then she can expect closer scrutiny, and this consideration should be included in the equation. She should make especially sure that she is armed with facts when making a presentation, and she should not reveal her emotions in public. Chiefs do not cry in public. Like her male counterpart, she should be careful with expressions of friendship, gratitude, or loyalty in private, lest they should be misinterpreted. At meetings of equals, dress and jewelry should be distinctive but not extravagant. Subdued elegance and exquisite taste may add to her effectiveness, but she should never be coy or flirtatious. Her presentations should be short and laden with data. Remember that even though the women executive has broken the glass ceiling, she may be using a leadership approach that differs from what many are used to.

In summary, the equal chiefs in companies or universities can be your most important allies in battle, and they generally will respond to collegiality, generosity, and your willingness to sacrifice your own unit's interests for the broader welfare of the company or university

HOW TO TREAT
SUBORDINATES

Share the fruits of success with your subordinates. Do not have favorites. Be visible and listen carefully to suggestions and complaints. Praise in public, chastise in private. Instill confidence and pride in the unit.

Subordinates can make or break the chief. How they function, and fulfill the chief's expectations depends on many factors, and important among them is leadership. Jack Welch, the chairman and former CEO of General Electric, is an excellent case in point. He took over a large, potentially stagnant company and made it into the envy of the whole world by making wise and bold decisions and inspiring everyone in the company. To achieve that end, he displayed in a most impressive manner what leadership is about: integrity, vision, the courage to take risks, superb taste in choosing associates, and, most important, the ability to mesmerize subordinates by paying attention to their contributions. His willingness to share the fruits of success with them generated true team spirit in a global company. In academia, Clark Kerr, the creator of the modern "multiuniversity" is another example. He obtained enthusiastic support from a notoriously cantankerous faculty and inspired them to create a state university based on several diverse campuses that could, through the quality of their research and education, match and surpass the nation's most prestigious private universities. In addition to further enhancing the prestige of UC Berkeley UCSF, and UCLA, he added several more campuses and allowed them to develop their own individuality while maintaining the highest quality in all. Both Jack Welch and Clark Kerr, though in different arenas, were using the same approach as that used by the military as far back as in the days of specially selected and named Roman legions and as recently as the era of special outfits in modern armies. The red, black, or green berets and the various airborne outfits in recent conflicts are examples. Naming a unit with an inspiring motto such as "The Screaming Eagles," "The Invincibles," or something similarly uplifting and assigning them a distinctive cap and shoulder patch instills pride. This pride leads to the high morale of winners who will go flat out for their outfit and never surrender, even at ultimate personal sacrifice.

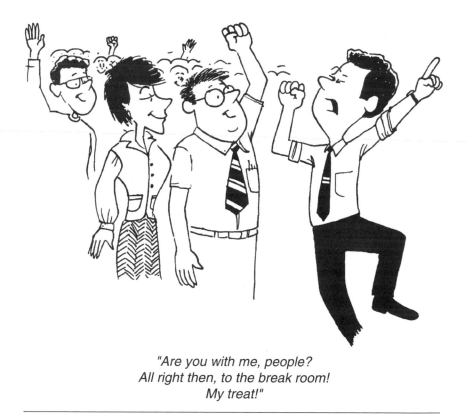

"Are you with me, people?
All right then, to the break room!
My treat!"

The leader of such an outfit in time of battle cannot sit in staff headquarters, safely far from the lines of combat, and expect to instill enthusiasm and a frenzied desire for victory. He must be on the first tank, like Erwin Rommell, George Patton, or Moshe Dayan to name only a few of the recent inspiring military leaders.

The mistake of not leading boldly and in full view is seen in stale, flabby, hierarchical organizations, where people are expending the least amount of effort—just enough to be acceptable for automatic promotions. The famous remark of Pope John XXVI is a good testimonial to this point. Guiding a distinguished visitor through the Vatican, who was impressed by the large number of prelates, bishops, and other high church dignitaries scurrying through the corridors with full briefcases, the visitor asked, "Oh my, how many people work here?" His Holiness answered coolly, "Roughly 50 percent."

In treating subordinates, the chief must constantly weigh opposing concepts: (a) The chief must be close to the subordinates in order to inspire them, learn about their suggestions, and hear their complaints; (b) simultaneously, the chief must be efficient by receiving information from close associates, producing plans for future actions, and supervising their execution.

The secrets for success are as follows

1. Create credibility.
2. Be visible and frank.
3. Back associates.
4. Be approachable.
5. When giving assignments, be clear. If there are choices to be made by the subordinate, define them with no ambiguity left.

Being visible means strolling through the department, offices, or factory in your domain and being willing to talk to the people there. A chief should not attempt to imitate the legendary caliph of Bagdad, Harun-Al-Rashid, or King Abdulah of Jordan and mingle with the subjects while in disguise in an effort to learn about the true state of the realm. A chief's position in modern business or academia is not sufficiently exalted for such exploits. Mingling, asking questions, and listening is, however, invaluable. A modern chief should also have a mailbox, solicit suggestions, acknowledge them, and even give prizes and recognition for the best suggestions.

Problems that come up may vary from complaints about safety to protests of discourtesy. Everything, even the silliest complaints, should be handled respectfully and, if need be, followed up on. In bad times, unpleasant cuts in pay or personnel may be inevitable. Design and implement justifiable, orderly, and equitable plans of how to proceed. It must be a method that your conscience can live with and that in spite of hardships to individuals does not destroy morale and create enemies for the enterprise. Be sure that you take the largest reduction in pay and benefits yourself, and make sure that everyone working for you knows this.

A head of a large university received a huge increase in salary and benefits that was published in that university's gazette at the same time that raises were frozen for everyone else. In fact, many employees were laid off at the same time, and there were other budget cuts. That the head's popularity and morale within the institution plummeted needs no elaboration.

Above all do not have favorites or close friends working for you. *The captain must be alone on the bridge.* If a member of your family or a relative of one of your closest associates starts working in the department that you head, make sure that someone else is in charge of that person. Remove yourself from supervision and make it clear to everyone that the rules applicable to everyone will be applied in spades. It may be a good idea, if possible, that your or your close associate's relative learns the ropes elsewhere. The obvious exception would be if you own the company and your successor and inheritor needs to learn about the company from the bottom up.

How should a woman chief treat subordinates in the outfit she heads? Her treatment should not be much different from that of her male colleague. She, however, even more than a man, should avoid being harsh and unpleasant. Women are generally believed to have more empathy than men, they tend to avoid confrontations, and have the ability to discipline with tact, which may be due to the more direct experience with parenting that many women have traditionally enjoyed. As they mingle with subordinates they have to learn to be distant yet friendly, interested without being prodding. Some women tend to show worries and anxiety about dealing with hard times. A woman chief must follow the same rule of demeanor applicable to men: Her consistent message should be that there may be difficult times ahead, but the staff members will be able to cope with them together and will emerge stronger and better; the chief has the answers but needs the backing of the staff. The refrain is the same: praise in public, chastise in private, and convey bad news the way you would most appreciate learning about it yourself. This approach will help to soften the blow and should be the immutable rule for all chiefs, men and women, if they wish to be respected and followed.

TREATING ADVERSITY

Never appear worried in public, yet do not appear overconfident and promise easy solutions. Do not cut resources so severely that vital functions are eliminated. Do not allow young, key members of the team to become discouraged and leave. Instill confidence that better times are coming.

If a chief has not faced adversity, he or she has been lucky, has had too short a tenure, or has failed to receive adequate information about the true state of affairs. With constant changes in economy affecting a business or university, bad times will surely occur. The maxim holds true: It is easy to excel when times are good, but it is in adversity that real leaders emerge. It is also much easier to command an advancing army than a retreating one. The latter requires great skill and fortitude, because in retreat it is easy to lose heart.

The chief who is a true leader instinctively inspires confidence.

The following maxim must guide you: Never appear worried in public, yet do not appear overconfident and promise solutions by repeating the unfortunate phrase used during the Vietnam War: "There is light at the end of the tunnel."

Work hard on plans that will get you out of trouble. If you are going to reduce the income of the people working in the unit, cut your own income and of those of your closest deputies most severely, and make sure everyone knows it. The harsh reality may be accepted more readily. Successful leadership depends heavily on symbols, examples, and never demanding from others what the leader is not willing to do himself or herself.

Some important guidelines are, however, very important:

1. No matter how difficult the conditions, do not cut resources so severely that vital functions are eliminated and you cannot recover full operations in a reasonable amount of time when the conditions change.

2. Hopefully, your plan for recovery should result in advancing beyond the point from which you had to retreat.

The following is an instructive story: A peasant was kneeling next to a ditch weeping over the carcass of his dead donkey. When bystanders asked what was going on, he replied, "Oh, unlucky me. Just when my poor donkey had learned to work without being fed, he went ahead and died on me." Do feed the donkey if you want him to keep working for you!

Avoid cutting vital resources and, equally important, do not let key employees go. Your most valuable team members must be reassured, their morale must be lifted, and they must be kept involved in planning for recovery. When recovery does occur, they must be given full credit. This is the best way to keep your employees from jumping ship.

Anyone who believes that he or she can do it alone and who does not listen carefully to criticism and advice is destined to become a loser. Once you and your organization have recovered, do not demand praise. You will only diminish your success. Victory speaks for itself and good leaders are expected to win.

How should a woman chief face adversity? No differently than a male chief. She should not be intimidated by the fact that her ship is in rough waters. More male chiefs fail than do female chiefs. These women are the chosen ones, with special qualities that made it possible for them to rise to the top. They generally are more able than their male colleagues and should remember Joan of Arc and Golda Meyer.

Being the chief is not always fun. It carries with it obligations, and the welfare of the outfit should guide all your decisions. Avoid strife, and if there are failures along the way, assume responsibility. If painful decisions have to be taken and top people have to be let go, do it yourself with compassion and tact. If you can transfer these people or find them a job elsewhere, do not delegate that task either. You have more chance of success than one of your subordinates. Do not feel sorry for yourself. Nobody promised you a bed of roses.

HOW TO RECRUIT AND
PROMOTE TALENT

*Select new recruits carefully and obtain reliable information
about their past performance. Do not let new appointees sink
or swim on their own. Give them increased authority in
gradual steps and be there when they need you. In recruiting,
you may be selecting your successor and relish that thought.
To be succeeded by someone as good or even better than you is
a great personal achievement. Promote on performance, not
on seniority.*

The high quality of your associates is the greatest asset that your unit
possesses. Their talent will guarantee the success of the subunits that
they are heading. Their sage advice and innovations will be responsible for
your and the whole unit's advances and possibly, in the business world,
survival. It is therefore essential to be a good judge of value when promoting within your own enterprise or recruiting from outside. To do so
successfully, you must obey certain basic rules:

1. Do rise above prejudices involving gender, race, sexual orienta-
tion, looks, background, or manners. Judge individuals entirely on the
basis of performance, ideas, originality, and integrity.

2. Evaluate past performance. People do not change once they are
adults. High performers will remain so, unless some personal or health
catastrophe changes them.

3. Gather information about future recruits carefully, directly, and
from reliable sources, and try to go back as far as possible.

4. Beware the possibility that another chief may be attempting to
"unload" someone that he or she wishes to leave.

5. Interview the applicant yourself and involve trusted associates in the evaluation.

6. Exchange impressions only after you have heard your associates' opinions. That will avoid your hearing only what they think you wish to hear.

7. If the individual that you wish to promote is within your own unit, and is exceptional, do not be swayed by the fact that his or her advancement will create jealousy, envy, and even some disturbance. Remember that President Franklin Delano Roosevelt promoted General George Marshall over many senior officers because of his promise, in spite of the fact that he was not even a West Point graduate, just a brilliant leader.

8. After being recruited for a high position from the outside or being promoted from within over the heads of seniors, do not leave the new appointees to sink or swim on their own. Nurture them, train them, give them increased authority in gradual steps, and be there when they need you.

Remember that you may be training your successor, and relish that thought. To be succeeded by someone as good or even better than you is a great personal achievement.

HOW TO LET YOUR
ASSOCIATES GO

The essence of letting associates go is to treat each case on its individual merits, and not allow emotions to influence your decisions. Take the long view, and do what is best for your unit and the people working for you.

Associates leave for three possible reasons:

1. They realize that they will be asked to do so and find other positions before the word spreads that they will be forced into mobility.
2. They are being transferred involuntarily within the company or university, or have been asked to seek a job elsewhere.
3. The associate is outstanding and has been recruited for a higher post elsewhere.

Because these situations arise almost daily, it is most advisable to discuss how to handle each without harming the enterprise and simultaneously keeping an eye on the future.

Situation 1. Individuals who are your associates must have an impressive background and have risen through the ranks on the basis of past accomplishments. The reasons they will eventually be asked to leave vary greatly. The most common is that, as in the Peter principle, they have risen and been promoted to the level of their incompetence. Another less common cause is that they and the modus operandi of the enterprise are no longer compatible. Perhaps the individual has become bored, exhausted due to the intensity of work, has unachievable expectations, or is dissatisfied with you. Family problems, divorce, illness, or the death of close relatives often are used as excuses for nonperformance. In any event, if the individual realizes that there is an imminent downward change in fortunes, do not feel guilty about the employee's decision to leave and do not try to persuade the person to change his or her mind and stay on. Encourage the employee to leave and talk only well about the past, emphasizing contributions he or she made before the employee's performance deteriorated. It costs you nothing to be magnanimous. It is important to be truthful but Delphic in the recommendation for an outside position. (Consider this example of a prophesy that the Delphi oracle in ancient Greece gave to a general before a battle: "If you cross the river with your army, events of decisive importance for you will follow!") In your letter of evaluation stress the good traits and past accomplishments that led to the employee's promotions; be very vague about failures and provide face-saving explanations.

Remember that to reach his or her present post, the incumbent must possess talent and be capable of good performance when the circumstances are propitious. Be particularly careful to avoid misrepresentations or exaggerations about the person's ability when talking or writing to friends who might employ this person. Presenting a loser as a winner to a friend is the surest way to spoil the relations, and the word will spread that your recommendations are not to be trusted. A famous scientist, when interviewing a potential hire, commented: "Your chief has written a great recommendation for you." Then after a short pause, "but your chief writes only glowing recommendations about everyone." After another pause, the scientist added, "He would not dare do that to me! You must be okay!" This exchange summarizes the caveats in writing recommendations. (The individual hired turned out to be a great success.)

Some very imaginative chiefs have devised a ruse that is usually successful. If they wish to get rid of an associate, they refrain from criticizing, pass the word that this superb individual is on the market, and appear hurt when he or she is being heavily recruited. Besides appearing chagrined, do nothing to match the outside offer and do not make any efforts to retain the associate.

Duplicity of this type must be reserved only for special cases, as the last thing a chief needs is to gain the reputation of being untrustworthy. When the individual is about to leave, just as you intended, do not be reticent about praising and giving dinners or other events honoring him or her. The individual's departure should be handled with dignity, and you will later find out that perhaps you did the individual an immense favor. Just do not go overboard. You and the departing individual know the truth.

Situation 2. An individual has to be let go or downgraded and possibly even sent to the equivalent of Siberia in your domain. What should you do? The best approach is to first make the decision about whether there is a future for the particular associate in your outfit. Determine whether he or she is salvageable or whether you are just avoiding hard decisions and possible confrontations if you keep him or her. Once you have decided honestly that a second, third, or even fourth chance is a waste of time, proceed by calling the individual into your office. Attempt to make the atmosphere as nonthreatening as possible. Inform the individual that in spite of the fact that you are asking him or her to leave, the person does have value. The circumstances are such, however, that you will have to insist that he or she leave or be significantly downgraded and sent to another job. Promise to keep your decision quiet for a while, which will assist to make it appear that the decision was made by the incumbent voluntarily. Also, you must set a time limit. There are two possible outcomes:

1. The individual will be successful in securing a satisfactory position elsewhere. In that case, there will be a send-off party and kudos.
2. The person will be unable to secure a new position elsewhere. The reasons could be (a) the true qualities (deficiencies) of the applicant are widely known, or (b) the individual has unrealistic expectations and demands too much.

What should you do in the case of event (b)? If there is a "Siberian" enclave in the company or university where the associate might be transferred, this is the most humane solution. The chief, however, must make sure that the individual brings value to where he or she is sent within the enterprise. If there is no "Siberia," or if there is one but you fear that the employee might bring the temperature there to an even lower point, give the associate a dismissal notice, specify the date of separation, and stick to it. It may be hard on you, but it must be done.

Situation 3. Suppose that a valued associate has decided to leave for greener pastures and a higher position elsewhere. You respect him or her, and the departure will result in significant loss to your unit. Ask yourself if you can match the offer in prestige, responsibilities, opportunities for advancement, or income. If the answer is yes, try to analyze why the individual even considered leaving. Were the conditions adverse? Were you too critical? Were you too stingy in praise or salary? Did you lose your temper? If the problem is correctable, do your best to change the conditions and ask the individual frankly what it would take to retain him or her. If you can afford to meet the demands, do so. If the demands are such that they would significantly threaten the intricate equilibrium that exists among other valuable equals in the unit, try to establish conditions that will be acceptable to both you and the associate, yet maintain peace in the unit. If the individual is so promising and exceptional that he or she is head and shoulders above the peers, disregard jealousies and offer the moon.

If the position offered elsewhere is advantageous to the individual and has all the attributes listed above that you must—more prestige, increased responsibilities, better opportunities for advancement and influence in the field, even satisfactory or better financial arrangements—and you have tried yet cannot match the offer, let the individual leave with your blessing and encouragement and keep him or her as a friend.

In academia it is one of the missions of a unit to produce leaders that will move and advance to other universities. This will make the field progress and will bring honor to your unit as one that consistently produces leaders. Try to be like the Benedictine abbey of Cluny. (In the tenth and eleventh centuries the French abbey of Cluny was reputed to be responsible for revitalizing and purifying the Catholic Church. At that time, the second sons of dukes and princes, when they became bishops and cardinals, behaved as if they were princes themselves—not as dedicated, pious churchmen. The abbots of Cluny, attracted, taught, and inspired the most promising novices in order to revitalize the church. In a short time, Cluny graduates became bishops, archbishops, cardinals, and even popes. Pope Urban II, who inspired the crusades, and Gregory VII, a great reformer, were graduates of that abbey). There is no greater honor than for a university to be known as the new Cluny in its discipline. Similar incubators of talent and centers of innovation happen also in industry. At one time almost every head of a large medical imaging company in the United States was a former associate of the legendary Walter Robb, head of General Electric Medical Systems, who was working for an even more famous company head, Jack Welch. Still, for an industrial company, the goals are different than they are for a university, and losing talent is more harmful. More effort must be expended to convince the brilliant associates to stay with the business. However, if nothing can be done to prevent the associate from leaving, accept the inevitable and put the best face to it.

The essence of letting associates go is to treat each case on its individual merits, not allow emotions to influence your decisions, take the long view, and do what is best for your unit and the people working for you. In business it is important to have contract clauses designed to limit the damage if an executive leaves to join a competing firm.

ENTERTAINING

*For whatever occasion, for whomever is entertained,
and regardless of where the activity takes place, do not give
up your own personal touch, taste, and dignity. Always
be true to yourself! Remember that every chief entertains
the way he feels most comfortable, expressing his or her
own taste.*

Entertaining means sharing one's privacy, time, and hospitality with other people. Depending on whether the chief is entertaining subordinates, equals, superiors, or other important guests, the rules change. They also differ depending on whether the people are to be entertained in the company or university building, in a restaurant or at home, or with or without spouses.

The most basic maxim about entertainment, is not to give up your own personal touch, taste, and dignity regardless of the occasion, site, or persons involved. Always be true to yourself! Remember that every chief entertains the way he or she feels most comfortable, expressing his or her own taste. The true noble tries to treat the guests as royalty, regardless of their station. The true measure of a prince or princess is to treat a beggar with as much politeness as the royal person would treat nobility. Let us consider each situation separately.

ENTERTAINING SUPERIORS AT A RESTAURANT

First of all, find out the taste of your guest, but also make sure, should it be very different from yours, that you find a compromise. There is no need to be uncomfortable by going to a restaurant or eating food that you despise, and certainly it is not proper to be lavish or extravagant. It is also inadvisable to go to a modest neighborhood restaurant in order to impress the superior about your frugality. Remember that your choice signals respect and thoughtfulness in selecting the ambience and cuisine that will please the individual and cater to his or her dietary restrictions. It also reflects your own taste. The latter is most important. You wish always to signal that you are secure and discriminating. Establish one or a few favorite restaurants where you will be recognized, remembered, greeted by name, and seated quickly. Waiting in a corridor or being sent to the bar where some members of your party may not even get a seat is unimpressive and can be embarrassing.

Private room dining is a no-no, unless there is a special celebration or business items need to be discussed. A private room may be a necessity only if the group having dinner is large and you require privacy. If the group is small, cocktails should be consumed at the table. Be careful about how much you drink. Try to stay with wine, and do not consume more than, at the most, two glasses during the whole evening. If your superior is a teetotaler, abstain out of respect, but do not make a show of it. For a party smaller than eight, have everyone order a la carte. For larger parties it might be advantageous to provide three fixed menu choices: meat (lamb or veal is what I would recommend), fish, or a vegetarian plate. This saves time and considerably simplifies ordering.

With one's business or university superior, there is no such thing as a purely social event. If the dinner is with spouses and a quasi-social occasion, try to keep the conversation flowing, particularly in the area of the guest's interest. This will require some discrete preliminary research. If the occasion requires you to mix some business with pleasure, try not to convey destructive news, and hope that your superior will not ruin the evening with something equally devastating for you.

The dress for the evening depends greatly on whether the dinner is right after work or if there is an intervening period of at least one hour. If the dinner is scheduled for right after work and you knew about it in advance, dress as if you wish to impress someone with your neatness. If you have time to change clothes in between work and dinner, a white or light blue shirt and dark (navy, charcoal gray, or black) suit with a contrasting but subdued motif necktie usually are perfect for men. For the woman executive, a dark suit (either with a skirt or pants) with elegant but not showy jewelry is a highly acceptable outfit.

Whether the dinner is with spouses or not requires important decisions. If dining with spouses, do not discuss business. Instead, try to make the evening as socially entertaining as possible. Seating is very important. Note that everyone in the room wants to sit either next to you or next to your superior. People who are assigned those seats of honor will not be particularly grateful to you, as they will feel that they deserve the honor. Those who sit near the periphery will feel slighted and resentful if they think that you have made these arrangements on purpose. A good prescription to avoid ruffled feathers is to mix guests as much as possible—a junior next to a senior, next to a junior, and so on. Deal similarly with the seating of spouses. Try to seat guests with shared interests next to each other.

The worst mistake you can make is to have the guest of honor and everyone "important" sit at one end of the table and all others of lower rank sit at the other end, which they will consider a form of exhile. Realize that usually not more than four people, and at maximum six, can participate actively in a conversation. Avoid and discourage a loud "lecture" to the group (unless it is being made by the guest of honor). Do not praise the restaurant or the food. If it were not outstanding, you would not have selected it. Praising either reveals insecurity or a desire to be reassured.

Dinners in the private dining room of your business or university should be reserved only for occasions when this is either convenient or symbolic. Never choose this site if you are entertaining your superior and if his or her office is located on the same campus or business site. This deprives you of your role as host.

ENTERTAINING SUPERIORS AT YOUR OWN HOME

Having your superior for dinner at your home requires careful orchestration, yet it must appear spontaneous and natural. Unless your spouse, you, and your superior and his or her spouse are celebrating a special, perhaps joint occasion, invite one and not more than two other couples who have interests and backgrounds that would make for an enjoyable and interesting evening. An important point is to have the event catered. Neither you nor your spouse should run around the apartment or house serving, refilling glasses, or removing dishes. Serving should be done quietly and efficiently. The conversation should not involve business, and the guests should be selected to make sure that there are no political, religious, or other clashes.

The meal requires meticulous planning and demands research about what the superior, the spouse, and the other guests like; you should certainly exclude what they hate or are not supposed to eat. Wines should be excellent but not ostentatiously expensive. Always offer after-dinner coffee and cordials. (Port, Armagnac, Cognac or liqueurs should be the choices. In cognacs try to offer X-O quality, Armagnac should have a vintage.) Never, never show videos or slides from your trips, unless you have made them together with the guests of honor, although even then the courteous approach would have been to have the videos or slides mailed at an appropriate, earlier time.

LUNCHES WITH SUPERIORS

Lunches are much simpler but still require a great deal of planning. Remember that the old two-martini lunch is distant history. Again, have it in your office if it is large enough or in the private business dining room if it is suitable. Select the latter site only if it is on your turf and not on your superior's. Whether in your office or in the business dining room, arrange for a simple lunch and, if possible, have at least two alternate choices. It is advisable to find out what your superior likes for lunch. Alcohol should neither be offered nor served.

A neighborhood restaurant may be an acceptable alternative. This shows that you value time, as you are not taking your guest to a renowned eating place far away. It is not advisable to have many people for such lunches, therefore everyone should order what she or he likes. As everyone will generally be expected to return to work in the afternoon, do not order a bottle of wine and certainly martinis or similar hard liquor are out. If the guest of honor insists, (or if he or she is European), have lunch in a restaurant that offers fine wines.

A lunch with your superior inevitably involves some business conversation. It is important, therefore, to have tables out of the earshot of others. If this is not possible, do not conduct business talk at the table. One never knows who is listening in. If you are seated at a secluded table or in a private dining room (which generally is not recommended unless your guest requests it) and if you are in charge of the agenda, avoid any discussion that may be painful. Have an optimistic, pleasant order of subjects, even if the painful items are reserved for after the meal.

ENTERTAINING EQUALS

Your approach need not change much when entertaining equals, except that this type of socializing almost never involves business. If it is business, then it is not entertaining and can be taken care of efficiently at lunch or in each other's office. If there is an agenda, if it will take longer than can be handled during a lunch, and if it needs to be connected to a dinner, you will most likely be responsible for the arrangements. Serve few or no alcoholic beverages during business lunches, and one should also limit alcohol consumption at business dinners.

When it comes to entertaining equals, there should be a difference in ambience if the evening dinner, or weekend lunch, is a celebration of some kind or if the get-together is a social repayment for a previous visit. Among equals there should not be any rules other than to share an enjoyable occasion that will bring the participants closer together. If there are income differences between you and your guest, do not make them felt, regardless of who is the wealthier. Always remember that equals can be important allies and that fostering friendships through entertaining should be natural and pleasant, whether at home, in a restaurant, at a country outing, or away from the city where you live. If you go out together often, share the bill. It avoids wrestling for the check and it prevents either party from feeling obligated and trying to remember who paid the last time out.

ENTERTAINING SUBORDINATES

This is more complicated than either entertaining superiors or equals. You may not be as aware of the differences in status as your subordinates are. There is no pretending. You can invite them either to a restaurant or your home for some special occasions, celebrations of some events, to present awards, or to give them a send-off to a higher position in your unit or elsewhere. Your guests will always feel that you are the boss. Be as friendly and natural as you can possibly be. Try to put your guests at ease, and by all means, if the celebration is taking place at your home, treat them as dignitaries. If you plan to go to a restaurant, choose a fine one but make sure that your guests are comfortable and not overawed. Do not banter or make jokes. Remember your subordinates cannot respond at an equal level.

In general subordinates are entertained as a group, either for traditional events, such as Christmas parties, celebrations of some special success of your entity, or special anniversaries. It is perfectly all right, even preferable, to have such an event in a restaurant or in the ballroom of a hotel. A hall in your company, if there is such space, or in a university building may be a suitable alternate choice. Such a locale even enhances the feeling of belonging to a select team. Usually such events are friendlier and more effective without spouses, as they generally are not involved in the daily contacts. However, there are exceptions. Some companies or university departments attempt to cultivate friendships of entire families. Such events are planned to include spouses, and sometimes even children are invited. The purpose of such mixing is to establish bonds. At all occasions that bring employees together, the chief should be among the first at the event, stay till the very end, mix, circulate, and be pleasant,

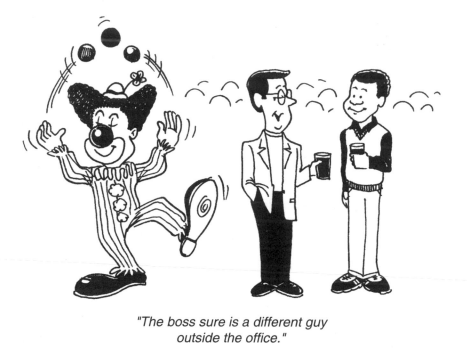

"The boss sure is a different guy outside the office."

complimentary, and upbeat. Try to remember names, but if you have difficulties to do so and if the department or business is large enough, perhaps it is not presumptuous to have name tags. Make sure the letters are in a large enough print for you to read the names as you talk to the individuals. Printing the first name in larger letters contributes to the atmosphere of cordiality. A common way of avoiding the perception of having forgotten a name that you should have remembered is to have the section in which the individual works also printed under the name. A very good approach is to exclaim, as you read the name, "Joe," or whatever the first name of the individual may be, "are you still in public relations? By now I expected you to be in the president's office," or something similarly light. Never be condescending, grave, or distant. Train yourself to be pleasant and friendly, and by all means appear at ease and natural.

ENTERTAINING AS YOU RECRUIT

Entertaining important recruits is a special art. Your participation should be reserved only for key positions, as otherwise you may not have any private life left and it will threaten peace in your family. Such entertainment is almost always done in restaurants and most everything that was stated about how to entertain superiors is applicable. You have to be the judge as to whether it is better to have more guests than only the recruit for lunch or dinner. If details of employment, salary, perquisites, and so on are to be discussed, only you and at utmost your deputy should be there. Write down or dictate for the record immediately, after lunch or dinner, what you have promised, as it is very easy to forget details. If recruitment arrangements have been made in your office, lunch or dinner should include your close associates and the recruit's important future coworkers. Spouses should be included for dinner only when the guest has been encouraged to bring his or her spouse.

Entreating at home during recruitment should be exceptional and reserved only for attracting individuals for the highest positions. Even then, there should be some special reasons why entertaining the recruit at your home is necessary or advantageous.

Occasionally, recruitment dinners or lunches follow negotiations at national conferences attended by you and the candidate. Entertainment should be in a restaurant and attended by your close associates if they are also at the conference. Spouses should be invited only if all in attendance are so accompanied.

ENTERTAINING IMPORTANT OUTSIDERS

Important guests that may be of value as customers, advisers, or (in the case of universities) large contributors should be entertained similarly to one's superiors with the exception that only rarely if ever would you entertain them at your home. Dinners at your home should be reserved only for close friends, and then the rules enunciated in the preceding pages do not apply.

Do not bore your important guests with tours of your business or university department, unless they have expressed special interest. Even then, make the tour short and comprehensive.

HAVING A NEW CHIEF

Do not give advice unless the new chief asks for it. If the new chief is friendly, be helpful but do not become a fixture in his or her office. If the new chief is hostile, examine whether you can fit in. You may decide that the changes are worthwhile and live with them. If you cannot get along, leave.

No matter how high your position in the company or university, you are bound to have a superior. It may be the president or chairman of the board in a company, the dean, chancellor, or university president in an academic setting, the editor-in-chief or publisher of a newspaper, and so on.

Even Jack Welch at General Electric—who was president, chairman of the board, and CEO in one person and thus theoretically had no superior—was always aware that, sooner or later, stockholders had to be pleased. But the concentration of power in his hands was an exception.

And remember nothing is permanent. Superiors change, get recruited away, retire, or even die.

Therefore, in whatever setting you function, the superior who recruited you or saw to it that you were promoted to the present post, the superior who delivered on his or her promises and kept praising you both in public and private, the person you could rely on, will eventually leave for one reason or another and will be replaced by a totally new individual. The new chief may be younger and more vigorous than the old chief, a person with his or her own predilections and plans for the whole entity, including your domain. You may feel that the new chief's ideas are based on prejudices. However, the new leader could be friendly or unfriendly to you and how you interact may make the difference between having a job that you enjoy, one that you despise, or not even having a job anymore at all. Remember that although you and your colleagues are nervous about the new chief, he or she is equally uneasy, as this is also a test for the newcomer.

HOW TO GET ALONG WITH A FRIENDLY NEW CHIEF

Anyone new, no matter how elevated the position, feels a little uneasy and unsure of him or herself. This is only natural, as getting one's bearings on a new position is of capital importance. No matter how well one is briefed, it takes personal assessment and reconnoitering before a new head of the enterprise can arrive at his or her own judgment on the state of affairs.

If it happens that what you have been doing matches the ideas of the new chief, and he or she feels that you are one of the entity's valuable assets, your life will be pleasant and you will enjoy the change. Do not assume, however, that this will last, and that you can from now on coast on your previous achievements.

The new chief will want a new beginning, new ideas that will distinguish his or her tenure from that of the previous chief. Based on your past performance you will be expected in business to do more with less and bring results that surpass those of before. In universities, your department is expected to win more competitive grants. You, and your associates will be expected to win awards, prizes, and medals, and to be elected to prestigious societies. You should be able to deliver all, as you are one of the inherited stars from the previous regime.

Although flattering, in many ways this expectation brings pressure with it as the ascending slope cannot go up forever. How is one to deal with these pressures?

1. Keep the chief informed and discuss your plans for the future with him or her. Schedule meetings as desired by the new chief, but do not become a fixture in the chief's office. Proximity diminishes respect.
2. Do not make your recommendations without careful discussions, submitted briefs, and plans from your associates and staff. Earlier chapters explored strategies for choosing your staff, and as before it is important to stress that the quality of the people on your staff is essential for success. Good taste in choosing associates is paramount.
3. Continue to act within you own domain as you did before the top management changed. You were successful before, and you should keep doing the things that made you so.
4. Do not give advice to the new chief, unless he or she asks for it. Refrain from patronizing or showing that you know the lay of the land better than he or she does.

5. Act naturally. Do not force contacts. After you have found out how the new chief wishes to operate the whole entity, cooperate and adapt without making obvious attempts to please. The latter only diminishes your stature.

6. Avoid social entanglements with the new regime beyond what is customary and sporadic. A respectful distance will be beneficial to all. Remember, the captain should be alone on the bridge. Your new chief should be given that privilege.

7. When asked to make a presentation, find out how the new chief wants it done. For instance, does he want preliminary handouts, summaries, or prints of the slides that you will show with your computer or overheads, or will the oral presentation itself suffice? Always be concise yet as informative as possible. Have the slides or computer presentation in color, with graphs and figures only if the new chief likes this type of presentation. Use as few images or graphs as necessary to make your points.

HOW TO GET ALONG WITH A HOSTILE NEW CHIEF

The new chief frequently has ideas about totally revamping the entity. His or her first impression may be that you do not fit into these plans. Your position may be shaky, although you have been highly successful in the past. You have, however, not been told that you should leave.

This is the time that you have to make the decision of whether to ride it out or quit. If you decide to quit, you may find that you actually did not have much choice in the matter. Do you find another position or do you retire? Retirement is feasible only if you have the financial reserves to maintain the desired living standard. Accepting a decline in living standards should be avoided if at all possible, as it is usually depressing, demeaning, and you will probably feel humiliated. Finding another position may not be easy, as the general rule is that good jobs become available when things are going well for you, but usually not when you sorely need them. Do not accept a new position just because you are desperate for a change. It could be, in effect, jumping from the frying pan into the fire.

It is likely that you have not thoroughly evaluated whether there is a chance that the situation in your present job could be turned around. It should be easier, unless you have been given notice, to find out how to get along with the new boss than to start elsewhere where you need to learn everything about new surroundings. The legendary success of Lee Iacocca at Chrysler after he was fired by Henry Ford II is an exception. This is so because Ford's dismissal of Iacocca was so patently capricious, public, and without a valid reason that it only raised esteem for the victim.

If you have the impression that the new chief considers you unable or unwilling to fit into the plans for revamping the enterprise, you should examine the plans that he or she may have presented. Try to be as unbiased as you can and determine in your mind whether they do fit into your set of values. You may come to the decision that it may be worthwhile to change the new chief's mind about you and cooperate with the new scenario. This, however, should be openly discussed, and, if possible, the two of you should reach an agreement about how you will fit into the new order. You may be surprised to find that things may work out and that you may actually agree with the changes that are being instituted, changes that perhaps have even been overdue. Just because you were comfortable with the old regime does not mean that it was good for the enterprise.

If you and the new chief reach an agreement about your staying on and cooperating, do not overreact.

1. Do the best you can to further the plans that you have agreed upon.

2. Do not try to endear yourself to the new chief. Be proper, friendly, and correct.

3. Avoid confrontations.

4. Have your plans for action carefully prepared, and present them in full detail before implementation. The presentation of your plan should be accompanied by a written or illustrated document. It is courteous to send it on before the presentation, to give the new chief a chance to study it in advance.

5. In meetings with colleagues of equal standing to yours in the enterprise, whether in the presence of the new chief or without him or her, do not criticize or voice opposition.

6. Realize that both you and your new superior are evaluating the new relationship, and until you have both firmly decided that you are to stay, every move is carefully weighed.

7. Life is too short for you to remain in an uncomfortable or possibly even humiliating position with a program you do not agree with or with a superior that you do not respect. Liking or not liking your new chief should not enter into the equation, but mutual respect is essential. Resign if you cannot stand the new situation. Do not act precipitously and attempt to get

a different job, as there is most likely no "golden parachute" in your contract. If properly handled, someone in the unit, perhaps even the new chief, may help you obtain a position elsewhere.

If you have decided to stay, the new chief has turned around, and you are being included in the plans for the future, the early negative relationship may resemble a distant nightmare. Perhaps after a period of time— once the cooperation has become almost automatic and mutual confidence has been established—the situation may become acceptable and even enjoyable. The early horror will, however, never be forgotten.

Much of this discussion refers to both businesses and universities. In academic life, however, there is a dichotomy between administrative and academic appointments. There is no tenure for administrative positions. In many universities in the United States, administrative performance is routinely reviewed every five to seven years. Some reviews are very thorough. The academic appointment with tenure, however, is for life. To avoid becoming a lost soul without the necessary skills to begin new academic pursuits, former academic chiefs need, and are often awarded, a sabbatical period for retraining. However, for many this is usually frustrating enough to lead to early retirement.

Women executives facing a hostile new chief are frequently confused, as it is not clear whether the negative attitude toward them is based on gender, previous record, qualifications, or personal incompatibility. Before you conclude on any of these, have it out frankly, as you will have to make very important decisions about your future. You may be surprised how an open exchange of plans and mutual expectations can clear the air. The plethora of lawyers in the United States has created an atmosphere of litigousness. Avoid involvement with lawyers who push for suits, unless there is an overwhelming reason for legal action.

RECRUITING

Do not promise more than you can deliver, but deliver more than you have promised. Rely on recommendations only from people you trust. It is an art to select top individuals and fit them into positions for which they are suited.

People are the most important ingredient of any enterprise. The quality of people, how they interact, how they fit into a program, and how they respond to leadership determines whether an entity will be successful. It is an art to select the right individuals to recruit, who will then accept the offer and join. Mentoring them to where they perform at their best, as well as independently is a vital follow-up. Successfully performing these functions is possibly among the most important attributes of a good leader.

It is axiomatic that to make good sausages you must start with good meat This certainly applies to recruiting. The difficult part is to have good taste and select the right individuals for the job to which they are best suited for. There are a few rules that generally work well in selecting the right candidates:

1. People do not change drastically. Steady, hardworking, high-quality performers began distinguishing themselves in elementary school and continued to do so throughout their schooling and post-scholastic employment.
2. Even late bloomers showed early achievements that were hidden under the cover of youthful rebellion.
3. Watch for continued signs of leadership. For instance, the person may have been school valedictorian, president of the class, chairman elected by peers of multiple councils, president of various professional groups, and so on.

4. Everyone, without exception, will have difficult periods in his or her life. Death of a beloved grandmother, a parent, or a sibling; parental divorce; the breakup of one's own marriage; disease—each of us will face some kind of challenge. They are common blows to one's equanimity. Find out the reaction that the candidate had to any of these challenges and whether the effects were detrimental to the individual's performance.

5. Carefully but discretely investigate the candidate's past performance from as early on as possible by directly contacting your friends and trustworthy colleagues. Unfavorable comments should not disqualify a person but should lead to a more thorough inquiry. Phone calls are much more valuable than letters.

6. The qualities you are looking for are (a) honesty, (b) truthfulness, (c) sincerity, (d) high intelligence, (e) originality, (f) leadership, (g) the ability to get along with peers, and (h) a willingness to work hard. Of all these, the first three are essential. A lack of or poor marks in any of these three qualities should be reason for disqualification. Encourage diversity if quality is equal. Diversity brings different experiences and additional viewpoints.

Candidates that possess all these positive qualities stand out and are prize subjects for recruitment. Do not be surprised that there is strong competition for such a candidate. You will need to be at your best to land the prized candidate. To do so, you need to have a program that will show that the following is true:

1. Your enterprise is among the best in the nation.

2. There is room for advancement to the top, although the present recruitment is at a somewhat lower level.

3. You, yourself, have a record for mentoring and promoting.

4. Many people that worked for you at the start of their career have been promoted.

5. There will be time for socializing, vacations, and bringing up a family.

Write the invitation for interviews letter yourself. Make it friendly and factual. Send a program along with information about the entity and about the position as well as about the job itself. If at all possible, greet the individual as the interviews start. Have everyone that sees the candidate call his or her impressions immediately to your executive secretary or to you. If everything is positive, offer the job, as you are the last interviewer.

Do not press the candidate for an acceptance. Allow him or her time for reflection. A generally uplifting remark that the candidates will remember forever is: "It is not for the job vacancy that we want you here. We want *You* for what you can contribute." A most important rule is this: *Never promise what you cannot deliver and try to deliver more than you have promised.* If you do this repeatedly, it will become part of your reputation and you will have few problems in recruiting.

It is a good strategy to hire a highly promising candidate to a position slightly lower than the eventual post that you hope the candidate will rise to. Promotions are always most encouraging. Should the candidate fail to meet all your expectations you can look for someone else without breaking any promises.

Rely heavily on recommendations about candidates from friends and colleagues from other institutions or companies as well as your own. Remember, close friends will not lead you astray because they will wish to preserve the relationship.

Beware of "dumping." A letter of recommendation from another department in the same university or another business unit in the same company that is attempting to transfer an undesirable individual should alert you to possible trouble. A recommendation such as "this person is so good, you should have her or him on your staff" could indicate an attempt to unload a problem employee.

During recruitment, introduce the candidate to the people she or he will work with at the same level and encourage bonding. Also introduce the candidate to the rising stars in the unit he or she is to head.

If the person you are recruiting is a woman and you are a man, the rules are basically the same. However, be very careful not to appear that you are flirting, and do not be overly familiar. Be careful that the questions you ask may be interpreted as too personal. The generally used custom of calling people by their first name is not the right approach until you become better acquainted or the candidate encourages you explicitly to use her first name. As mentioned in the chapter on how to use one's office, the woman recruit should be asked to sit in a chair at your office table, never on a couch, and certainly not with both of you sitting on the same couch. This is a prescription to make the candidate uncomfortable and ill at ease.

If the chief doing the recruiting is a woman, her behavior should be no different than that of a man. Avoid being "motherly" to a male candidate, and do bond with a woman whom you are recruiting. Avoid making confessions about the difficulties you have conquered. Do not appear to enlist the female recruit into the war of liberated women against the "man-dominated world."

PROMOTION TO THE NEXT STEP OF CHIEF

Avoid promotion to your level of incompetence. Do not let your promotion estrange you from your family.

S uccessful chiefs will undoubtedly be offered promotion to a higher position. This is particularly true if they have fixed long-standing problems, made their unit modern, efficient, and profitable if this is a business, or, if a university, led a laboratory or department in successful research with grants, achieving ground-breaking discoveries with trainees who later obtained important positions. The promotion offered can be to become the CEO or COO in a company, the dean or president in a university, or the president of an important national foundation. These promotions present a great challenge. It is important not to jump at the opportunity but to give it careful scrutiny and systematically review all the pros and cons. Do not be seduced by the glitter of flattery. Although each situation is different and the details of the promotion should be paid meticulous attention, many issues are generic and can be dealt with in general terms.

THE PROS

The pros of accepting a promotion are obvious:

1. You will get an opportunity to change the culture of the enterprise and make it more successful.
2. Recognition, more visibility, a larger staff to perform the mundane tasks, and a higher income generally go with the promotion and are powerful incentives.
3. The ability to have your favorite plans finally come to fruition is certainly attractive.

4. More freedom to make decisions and choose associates would be a dream come true.

5. If the company is large enough or the university is sufficiently prominent, your promotion may lead to national or international recognition.

6. The government or even the country's president may ask you for advice.

7. You may be invited to address international gatherings, like the world business leaders meeting in Davos, Switzerland.

8. You may be quoted in newspapers, interviewed on television, and treated like royalty.

9. Every pronouncement that you make will be quotable and you will be expected to spend a considerable fraction of your time on interviews, banquets, and basic public relations.

10. If you are very high in a university (dean, senior vice president, or president), you will also be expected to mix with the very wealthy in order to raise funds, with politicians to have the legislature or Congress pass appropriations favorable to your university and even with artists who are to perform in fund-raising events.

11. At banquets, whether your enterprise is the organizer or it is a public event, you and your spouse will be seated either at the head table or at the reserved table number 1, and you will be rubbing elbows with other notables and their spouses.

All this is exhilarating, inebriating, and your spouse may enjoy it. If you are able to keep the relationships with your family, spouse, and children warm and unaffected by your rise to prominence, the experience will be enjoyable for all. This is especially true if you are able to mix business with pleasure when you travel and take your spouse and sometimes also your children with you.

THE CONS

Almost every statement made in the section on pros has its counterpoint. The basic question to be answered after careful analysis is this: Is this promotion a confirmation of the Peter Principle (which states that one gets promoted to his or her level of incompetence)? In other words, examine whether the position you are being offered is one in which you can be as successful as you have been in your current position. Remember that the higher you reach, the less you will actually be in control over the immediate turn of events in the field.

One example can be provided by an army in combat. The commander of an army or army group will be in contact with the corps and division commanders by scrambled radio signals. The commander's basic involvement will come from moving little flags on the map. On the other hand, an airborne division commander will be commanding troops in the field and will be in direct contact with the situation. If this commander wishes to make a decision without checking with the army commander, he or she can get away with it by claiming that contact has been lost! Heading a branch of the business, or a university laboratory or a department gives you similar freedom and control and even fulfillment. Be aware that this may be lost when you assume the top position.

Being quotable also has downsides. Every comment that you make, even in private, will be quotable. The higher your post, the less likely it is that what you say will be considered "off the record." Your conversations at restaurants may be overheard by people you have never met and who will love to quote you. Some of your statements will be exaggerated, distorted, and taken out of context, as news is more appreciated if it is sensational. For example, a highly respected preacher started his sermon with the thunderous exclamation, "There is no God, atheists and sinners would make you believe." Quoting only the first four words will draw attention, but this is the opposite of what the preacher said.

Not having privacy gets old in a hurry. Sitting at the head table or table number 1 often means being with uninteresting snobs. It would be fun to sit, once in a while, with truly interesting but not powerful people whom you enjoy. Furthermore, going out all the time and being a public figure requires a special type of personality. Examine yourself as to whether or not you fit into the mode of the new position.

Do not neglect your family. It is easy to be so overwhelmed by day-to-day problems that you come home later and later. Before you know it, you become estranged from the ones whom you love most: your spouse and your children. There are so many examples of divorces of "successful" people and of children of powerful people getting into serious trouble, making this discussion superfluous. Sometimes being promoted to the higher position may require relocating. This may require your spouse to leave his or her job as long-distance marriages usually do not last. The children may balk initially. You will be taking them out of their schools and separating them from their friends. Even if they are in college, coming home will be different. So think about it before you accept a promotion. Remember also that except for the summit positions with Joseph Stalin, there are very few lifetime top jobs. There is a "life after," which should also be considered. Descending from the summit of power can be traumatic.

SURVIVING AWAY FROM THE JOB

There is life away from your work. Try to enjoy it with those close to you. Relaxing away from the job will make you more effective at it.

Unless you are made of steel, stress at work will sap your energy and tend to make you feel that you are in a pressure cooker. No matter how efficient you are, work never seems to be completed and you are always behind. Get used to it. Unless your administrative assistant is an exception and knows how to say no to many people, your appointment schedule will be full to the brim every day. You may not even have time to think between meetings. You drive or are driven home, always late and usually, particularly if you are in the back seat of the car, making more calls on the cellular phone. You come home and if you have had a bad day at the office you are preoccupied, short tempered, and basically not fun to be with for your spouse or children. After dinner, you will probably still ruminate about the bad day that you have had, about the plans that will have to be finalized tomorrow, and about why things don't go more rapidly and smoothly. After you twist and turn, you finally fall asleep and frequently have nightmares.

Is there a way out? I do not believe that psychologists or psychiatrists can be of help because your behavior is within the normal range for an executive, and your reactions are those that most people in your position experience. To make life and your successes enjoyable, you must train yourself to adhere rigorously to the following tenet: Once the door of your office is closed, you must not think about your job. You should focus on your social life, vacations, family obligations, personal purchases, and so on. Otherwise you will not acquire peace of mind. The separation of job and private life is essential but not easily achieved. It takes discipline and a strong will to stop thinking about work and job-related problems.

Try to listen to the news or your favorite music on the way home. When you arrive there, start the evening with a glass of champagne or wine with your spouse. Ask about what is new in the household. If your spouse also has a profession or a job, inquire what is new there. But at least for the evening, do not talk about your job and issues related to it. There is so much happening in the world that one can talk about: politics, theater, books, children, neighbors, vacations. As the evening progresses, the job-related problems will fade into and meld with those of the rest of the world, and they will assume their proper significance. Falling asleep may be difficult, as thoughts about work do not recede easily. One of the most successful ways to fall asleep is to keep telling and repeating to yourself, "Stop right now and fall asleep." Block all other thoughts. It is unbelievably simple, but it works.

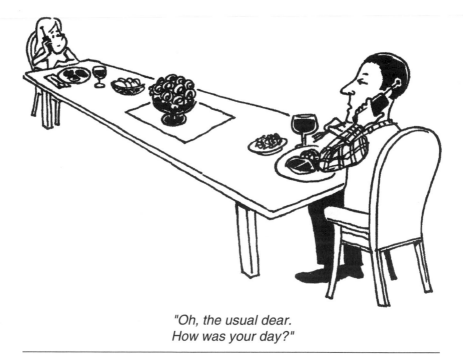

"Oh, the usual dear.
How was your day?"

While this prescription for arriving home and resting after dinner works for some time, the monotony of repetition after a while takes its toll and you may need alternate ways of achieving peace of mind. Dining out with just your spouse is one. Weekend trips help. Vacations to places that everyone in the family likes offer a great way to rest and recuperate. Also take trips to conventions and to meetings of groups that you enjoy. Physical fitness is important. Try to exercise every day. For a busy person, mornings before breakfast are the best time for exercise, as during the day you are probably too busy. While it is true that nothing will be lost if you go to the gym for half an hour, that half hour of exercise just will not happen. Select a sport that you enjoy. If your spouse likes the same sport, do it together but do not compete against each other. All this does not preclude your love for your job, Your job, however, should not exclude everything else from your life.

_____ SAYING GOODBYE

Retirement is a reminder that everything, even life, is temporary. Do not grieve, but if you are in good health and in possession of your wits, enjoy life with dignity and be proud of past glories.

All things in life—good, bad, or indifferent—must end sooner or later. Your position, no matter how elevated, will end unless you own the business. Even then there must be a time when leadership should be transferred to someone younger with more vigor and fresh ideas appropriate to the times. This should hopefully occur before you or those closest to you feel that your judgment is failing.

IN A BUSINESS

In a business, the end of your tenure may come with retirement, with your own decision to leave the company, or by being asked to resign. While there may be variations of these three general modes, the unalterable fact is that you are leaving the position that you have had and your leadership of the enterprise has come to an end.

If you retire, you will have some great memories. However, retirement is itself a reminder that everything, even life, is temporary. This adds a bittersweet flavor to the event. There will be multiple recognition and well-wishing dinners and gatherings with speeches, gifts, and books with letters of appreciation from employees and coworkers. Most will be sincere and heart warming. Your colleagues will probably also give you a dinner with roasting and most likely with some ribald jokes unless you are a woman. If you have been particularly successful, your portrait in oil will be hung in the headquarters of the business in a hall or the boardroom.

IN A UNIVERSITY

If donors can be recruited and motivated, a chair may be endowed in your name. If you have greatly impressed a billionaire, a building, hall, or amphitheater might be named after you. A lectureship in your name, honoring your tenure as chief, generally is an indication that the donors were not generous enough for an endowed chair in your name. Getting sufficient funds from members of your laboratory or department is difficult, even for a lectureship, unless it is marked only for one or two repetitions of the event. Funds from various contributors to honor your tenure will be more generous if solicited before the end of your tenure, while you are still in power. This is because as time passes after you have retired, no matter how famous or loved you were, the memory of your contributions will fade. Discretionary funds are rarely used for this purpose.

Do not believe, however, that the remembrance of your successes will be enhanced by all these mementos. If the gifts are large enough to name a building, hall, or endowed professorship in your name, a few years after you are gone, everyone will believe that you were a generous, rich industrialist, banker, or a less well known philanthropist. If you were very successful and someone has contributed funds for the painting of your portrait, it may be hung in a hall or corridor in the university, unless your successor carries a grudge and vetoes it.

Do not be surprised if you telephone your former office and a new secretary asks you to spell your last name. This happened to one of my former chiefs, a famous department head in retirement, who entered the waiting room in front of his former office and asked the new receptionist to announce him to his successor. The receptionist asked my friend to repeat his name. It was all the more ironic that she was sitting under his portrait!

HOW TO BEHAVE AT THE GOODBYE DINNERS, RECEPTIONS, OR GATHERINGS IN YOUR HONOR

Undoubtedly there will be toasts, speeches glorifying your achievements and contributions, exaggerations about your successes, and exclamations that you will never be forgotten. Remember that these are customary rites and that you have attended many similar ceremonies yourself. Therefore, remember that chiefs don't cry! But it is impressive and touching if everyone can see mist in your eyes. That is a sincere, telling sign of appreciation. Your expected remarks should be mercifully short, self-deprecating, and, if you can manage, witty and funny. But do not ridicule anyone except, gently, yourself. By all means, do not verbally attack anyone, even by pretending that it is in fun. Do not visit your former office for at least a year, even if you live across the street.

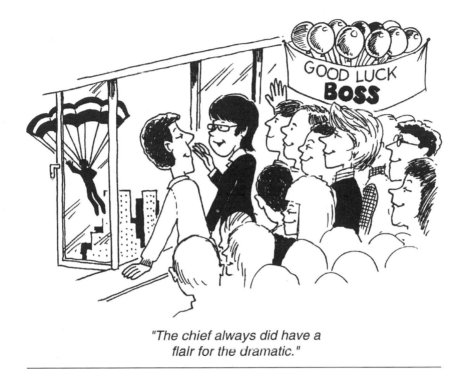

*"The chief always did have a
flair for the dramatic."*

If you retired from an administrative executive position in a university, and if you still have the skills you used in your professional life before becoming an administrator, go back to laboratory research, clinical practice, teaching, or lecturing, as you did previously. Do not ever interfere with the administration of your successor. Be happy and satisfied that you can still be useful as an emeritus. The ending in business is similar to the retirement in European universities. The cutoff is sudden and final. You hear the door slammed loudly behind you.

YOU ARE MOVING TO ANOTHER JOB ELSEWHERE

The customs followed if you move onto another job are the same as those that apply for retirement, unless you are making a lateral movie to head a competitor organization or university. If this happens, instead of the goodbye festivities, your administrative assistant and your close friends in the company or university may invite you for lunch. The temperature of relations with the rest of the members in your old entity will approach freezing. At the small gatherings, you do not need to exhibit the same emotions as if you were retiring and the toasts will also be less elegiac. Well wishers, however, will be more flattering as, who knows, perhaps in the future, you may recruit them to your new fief, and to a higher position than they now occupy.

IF YOU ARE ASKED TO RESIGN

The expression "success has many fathers, failure is an orphan" holds true. Even if close friends in the business hold dinners in your honor, in defiance of the decision to let you go, think twice about attending. You will wish to leave as quietly as possible and not cause problems and display unhappiness. Leaving without public recriminations may actually be part of the "golden parachute" agreement that you should have negotiated.

In a university, you most likely have tenure, making it possible for you to return to your area of expertise. If your professorial skills have cooled off, you may reheat them with a sabbatical leave. If that is not possible, you may still be eligible to head a charitable foundation, become editor of a journal, write books, or even enjoy a leisurely life in semiretirement, writing, reading, and lecturing. Grieving is an unnecessary self-torture if you are in good health, in possession of your wits, have an income sufficient to live in dignity, and are able to pay your bills. Be proud of past glories!

EPILOGUE: SURVIVING AND ENJOYING RETIREMENT

The most important part of a successful retirement is to transform it into a new, exciting phase of life.

The music is over, the celebrants have gone home. You are left with your memories, and the task is to make your life as pleasant as possible.

How do you arrange your retirement to make it pleasant and enjoyable? That you have a pension plan, savings, a home, and perhaps even a vacation second home is almost always true. If you have prepared your financial security, you have one less issue to worry about.

Retirement should be an enjoyable, relaxing, yet exciting phase of one's life. This is especially so today, with advances in medicine and surgery that allow a normal and functional life span to extend often into the ninth or even tenth decade.

Do not neglect your health. Spend the time and money necessary to have yourself medically screened on a periodic basis. Discovering a disease early usually makes treatment easier and generally more successful. If your health permits it, have that knee or hip replaced in order to live a normal, mobile existence.

However, no matter what you used to do, do not allow retirement to surprise you without your having made plans to enjoy it. Preparation is needed no matter what your background may be. If you have hobbies in which you could not fully engage while you were working full time (like collecting antiques or art, composing music, writing, going to concerts or the theater, or traveling), this is the time to enjoy them. Writing memoirs generally is not a good idea. If you are going to be totally frank about people with whom you have dealt, the book should be published only posthumously, which is not inviting, unless you are vindictive. A book based on your experiences, analyzing mistakes that you have made and becoming a morning-after quarterback with suggestions on how you might have corrected them is only a slightly better idea. Writing about your life without referring to business experiences may be enjoyable.

To many, descending from the peak of power to the fear of becoming insignificant is traumatic. The best way to prevent becoming depressed is to avoid meeting people who have been accustomed to seeing you in power as they may be condescending, or you may be interpreting their behavior as such. Attempt to start a totally new and exciting life, away from the site where you have been known as an important executive. Read, listen to music, go to theaters, play as many sports as your physical condition will allow, travel, and develop a closer relationship with your spouse than you may have been able to maintain while working at your job. Avoid interfering with your spouse's favorite schedule. The saying I married you for better or worse, but not for lunch is a message to be listened to.

However, if you enjoyed the kind of work you did before and want to continue doing it in some capacity, you may wish to become a consultant, perhaps to the government (avoid conflicts of interest), with or without remuneration. You can get involved in charitable work and find it highly rewarding. If you like it, volunteer. But do it part time, never full time. It is so easy to find yourself harnessed. You will not be able to understand how this could have happened to you.

If you enjoy politics, running for city council or school board in your suburb or city (never in a metropolis) may be fun. But this is true only if you do not get infected by the ambition bug, decide that you want to save the world, and start seriously running for a big political office. Make your contribution limited in time and do it purely as a public service, your way of paying back society. Do not go overboard.

The most important part of a successful retired life is to make it fresh and exciting. Enjoy it, be active, and do not make it into the phase where you are waiting for the inevitable end. The end will come, whether we are waiting for it or not. When it arrives, looking back you should be able to feel that, unlike Dr. Faust, you have had it all without having to trade your soul for the joys of your career and a full life.

References

BENTON, D. A. *Lions Don't Need to Roar.* Warner Books, New York, 1992.

BLANCHARD, KENNETH, and JOHNSON, SPENCER. *The One-Minute Manager.* Harper Collins, Hammersmith, London, 1996.

CARLSON, RICHARD. *Don't Sweat the Small Stuff.* Hyperion, New York, 1997.

COLLINS, JAMES C., and PORRAS, JERRY I. *Built to Last.* Harper Collins, New York, 1997.

COVEY, STEPHEN R. *The 7 Habits of Highly Effective People.* Fireside Edition, Simon and Schuster, New York, 1990.

FAST, JULIUS. *Body Language.* Pocket Books, New York, 1971.

FISHER, ROGER and URY, WILLIAM, *Getting to Yes. Negotiating Agreement without Giving In.* Penguin Books, New York, 1981.

GARDNER, JOHN W. *On Leadership.* The Free Press, New York, 1990.

GROVE, ANDREW S. *Ony the Paranoid Survive.* Doubleday, New York, 1996.

HAYWARD, STEVEN. *Churchill on Leadership: Executive Success in the Face of Adversity.* Primsa Publishing, Forum Rocklin, CA, 1997.

HEIM, PAT. *Hardball for Women.* Penguin Books, New York, 1993.

HOWAR, PHILIP K. *The Death of Common Sense.* Warner Books, New York, 1996.

LOWE, JANET. *Jack Welch Speaks.* John Wiley & Sons, New York, 1998.

MACHIAVELLI, NICOLO. *The Prince.*

MAXWELL, JOHN C. *The 21 Irrefutable Laws of Leadership.* Thomas Nelson Publishers, Nashville, TN, 1988.

MORONE, JOSEPH G. *Winning in High-Tech Markets.* Harvard Business School Press, Boston, 1993.

MUNDY, LINUS. *Slow-Down Therapy.* Abbey Press, St. Meinard, IN, 1990.

PARKINSON, NORTHCOTE C. *Parkinson's Law.* Bucaneer Books, Cutchogue, NY, 1957.

PETER, LAURENCE J., and HULL, RAYMOND. *The Peter Principle.* William Morrow & Co., London, 1969.

PETERS, TOM. *Thriving on Chaos.* Video Publishing House, Schaumburg, IL, 1987.

PHILLIPS, DONALD T. *Lincoln on Leadership.* Warner Books, New York, 1992.

SUN-TZU. *The Art of War.* Translation by Roger Ames. Balantine Books, New York, 1993.

WATERMAN, ROBERT H., JR. *The Renewal Factor.* Bantam Books, New York, 1987.

WECHSBERG, JOSEPH. *The Merchant Bankers.* Little Brown & Co., Boston, 1966.

WILSON, MIKE. *The Difference between God and Larry Ellison.* William Morrow and Co., New York, 1997.

WILSON PRICE, MARJORIE, and MCLAUGHLIN, CURTIS P. *Leadership and Management in Academic Medicine.* Jossey-Bass, San Francisco, 1984.

Leaders Interviewed

ALBRIGHT, CLARICE Former Director, Memorial Hospital; Owner, 2nd Reef

BASS BAKAR, BARBARA Former CEO, I Magnin; Member, Multiple Company Boards

BISHOP, MICHAEL Nobelist, Chancellor, UCSF

BRODY, WILLIAM President, Johns Hopkins University

FRITSCHE, PEGGY President-Elect, RSNA; Owner, Imaging Center

GOLDBERG, JANICE Owner, Delicious Catering, San Refael, CA

GUNN, JOHN Executive Vice President, MSKCC; Member, Multiple Company Boards

IMMELT, JEFFREY R. Chairman of Board, President and CEO, General Electric Corp.

KAUFMAN, LEON Former VP, Toshiba; CEO, Accuimage

KORN, PHILIP Former VP, Purchasing and Distribution, General Foods

KREVANS, JULIUS Former Dean and Former Chancellor, UCSF

LISSNER, JOSEF Former Chair, Radiology, University of Munich; Founder, European Congress of Radiology

MARKS, PAUL Director of Memorial Sloan Kettering Cancer Center, Emeritus

MILLER, GARRY CEO, First People Company, San Diego

REISER MAXIMILIAN Chairman, Department of Radiology, Ludwig-Maximillian University of Munich; President, German Radiology Society

ROBB, WALTER Former President, GEMS; Former Senior VP, GE Research; Multiple Company Boards

SMITH, LLOYD HOLLINGWORTH (HOLLY) Leader American Academic Medicine; Former Chair Department of Medicine, Associate Dean, School of Medicine, UCSF

SPAULDING, BRUCE Vice Chancellor, UCSF

STERN, HOWARD Executive Chairman of the Board, EZ-Em

WALL, SUSAN Associate Dean for Education, School of Medicine, UCSF

ZERHOUNI, ELIAS Executive Vice Dean, Chair Radiology, Johns Hopkins School of Medicine

Index